SENSE-PERCEPTION AND MATTER

Founded by C. K. Ogden

The International Library of Psychology

COGNITIVE PSYCHOLOGY
In 21 Volumes

SENSE-PERCEPTION AND MATTER

A Critical Analysis of C D Broad's Theory of Perception

MARTIN LEAN

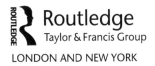

Routledge
Taylor & Francis Group

LONDON AND NEW YORK

First published in 1953 by
Routledge
2 Park Square, Milton Park, Abingdon, Oxfordshire OX14 4RN
711 Third Avenue, New York, NY 10017

First issued in paperback 2014

Routledge is an imprint of the Taylor and Francis Group, an informa business

© 1953 Martin Lean

British Library Cataloguing in Publication Data
A CIP catalogue record for this book
is available from the British Library

Sense-Perception and Matter
ISBN 0415-20964-1
Cognitive Psychology: 21 Volumes
ISBN 0415-21126-3
The International Library of Psychology: 204 Volumes
ISBN 0415-19132-7

ISBN 13: 978-1-138-87498-5 (pbk)
ISBN 13: 978-0-415-20964-9 (hbk)

CONTENTS

PREFACE

THE present essay is an abridged and slightly revised version of a study originally written in 1944–45, when I was in residence for the doctorate degree in philosophy at Columbia University. It was my good fortune to be in residence while Professor G. E. Moore was Visiting Professor from Cambridge University. In his lectures and in the departmental seminars, in which he vigorously participated, Professor Moore devoted considerable attention to puzzles about 'our knowledge of the external world'; and it was he who resolved my search for a suitable dissertation topic by suggesting a careful, piecemeal examination and criticism of C. D. Broad's argument in Chapter IV of *The Mind and Its Place in Nature* concerning 'Sense-Perception and Matter'. Although it cannot be gainsaid that I have followed his recommendation as to topic and approach, I cannot hope to have met his standard of carefulness. Unfortunately he returned to England before I was able to submit my efforts to his criticism. None the less, while the underlying viewpoint differs from his in important respects, it should be said that I am indebted to him for many of the ideas in this essay, however badly I may have handled them.

In the actual writing, my indebtedness is first and foremost to my teacher, Professor Ernest Nagel. For his invaluable guidance and criticism, for the generosity with which he gave of his time and attention, and for his intellectual tolerance and kindly encouragement throughout, I wish to express my deepest gratitude. I should like also to thank Professors Herbert W. Schneider, Irwin Edman, and Justus Buchler for their helpful criticisms and suggestions. And to *all* my former teachers in the Department of Philosophy at Columbia University I want to express my sincere appreciation for the award of a University Fellowship, which enabled me to pursue my studies and to write the dissertation; for the subsequent award of the Woodbridge Prize, which led to this publication; and above all for the stimulus of their teaching and of their intellectual company.

For the genuine help they provided in the crystallization of the ideas presented in this essay, I want to acknowledge the frequent discussion and argument of the issues which I enjoyed with my good friend Dr. John Hospers, when we were students together at Columbia University. Thanks are due also to Professors A. J. Ayer and Max Black for their kindly interest and for their generosity in having taken the time and trouble to look over the manuscript and to offer some encouragement along with valuable critical comments. And to my good friend Mr. C. D. Rollins I am particularly indebted both for his careful reading and constructive criticism of the manuscript, and for his help and encouragement regarding its publication.

While it would be impracticable to mention here by name all the philosophers from whose views my own most directly stem, anyone familiar with the so-called linguistic movement in contemporary philosophy, and particularly with the writings of those whose primary concern is with the logic of ordinary language, will recognize the extent to which the ideas expressed in this essay reflect theirs. Specific mention ought to be made, however, of the basic influence of my friend and former teacher at the University of Nebraska, Professor Oets K. Bouwsma, from whom I gained my earliest insights into the nature of language and its relation to philosophical problems.

Finally, it should be said that partly owing to practical circumstances—not the least of which was the pressure of time—and partly to philosophical disagreement, I was not always able to act upon the criticisms and suggestions which I sought and received in the writing and editing of this volume. Though I am not the less grateful, it follows that I alone must assume responsibility for all the respects in which it may be vulnerable.

M. L.

BROOKLYN COLLEGE
BROOKLYN, N.Y.
October, 1952

ACKNOWLEDGMENTS

FOR generous permission to quote from the copyright works indicated, acknowledgment and thanks are due to the following publishers:
Routledge & Kegan Paul Ltd.: *The Mind and Its Place in Nature* and *Scientific Thought* by C. D. Broad, and *Tractatus Logico-Philosophicus* by Ludwig Wittgenstein; George Allen & Unwin, Ltd.: 'Critical and Speculative Philosophy' by C. D. Broad, and 'A Defence of Common Sense' by G. E. Moore (in *Contemporary British Philosophy*, J. H. Muirhead, ed., first and second series, respectively); Tudor Publishing Co., N.Y.: 'A Reply to My Critics' by G. E. Moore, and 'Moore's Technique' by J. Wisdom (in *The Philosophy of G. E. Moore*, P. A. Schilpp, ed., The Library of Living Philosophers, vol. 4); Oxford University Press: *The Problems of Philosophy* by Bertrand Russell (in the Home University Library); Robert M. McBride & Co., N.Y.: *Perception* by H. H. Price.

INTRODUCTION

'One must be very brave to go against common sense.'
'Yes, and a fool as well.'

(Dostoievsky, *The Possessed*)

THERE is a type of approach to the analysis of our perceptual knowledge of physical objects which has led philosophers, past and present, to the very remarkable conclusions that we cannot with any certainty *know* that such objects exist, and that, if they do, their nature must be quite different from what it is commonly conceived to be. This approach is known in present-day philosophy as *sense-datum analysis*.

A leading contemporary exponent of this procedure and of these remarkable conclusions is Professor C. D. Broad, of Trinity College, Cambridge. In his various epistemological writings Dr. Broad employs the sense-datum approach in the form of an argument designed to show the untenability of our common-sense notions about physical objects and perception. In the present essay I have subjected this argument to a critical examination, the object of which is to defend these common-sense notions.

Although views essentially similar to his, in some or all of the respects important to my argument, have been advanced by many philosophers—Locke, Berkeley, Hume, Moore, Russell, to name but a few—the detailed exposition and criticism in the main body of this essay will deal directly only with Dr. Broad's presentation. For I want thus, by the intensive analysis of a single clear and concise formulation, to show just how the supposedly 'neutral' sense-datum approach actually *produces* scepticism and paradox about 'our knowledge of the external world', and also the extent to which the whole problem may be averted or dissipated simply by critical attention to the language in which it is generated.

In this essay I have no 'theory', philosophical or otherwise, to present in substitution for those which Dr. Broad advances. The thesis throughout is, rather, that the problems which he raises and for which he proposes these 'theories' are *pseudo-problems*, of a verbal as opposed to material sort. The truth is, I maintain, that we are already quite familiar with the salient empirical facts necessary to understand the nature of perception, so far, at least, as 'our knowledge of the external world' is concerned. And any *philosophical* 'theory' about it can be no more than a verbal reformulation of these facts.

Dr. Broad's treatment of the phenomenology of sense-perception has, over the years, exhibited a growth in complexity and subtlety ranging from the relatively elementary presentation in his *Perception, Physics and Reality* (1914), to the highly sophisticated account in his most recent major opus, the *Examination of McTaggart's Philosophy* (Vol. I, 1933, and especially Vol. II, 1938). But the most exhaustive and detailed account of his own views on perception and matter, and of the arguments which he advances in support of these views, as against common sense, is to be found in his *Scientific Thought* (1923) and in *The Mind and Its Place in Nature*[1] (1925). It is with the treatment in these, and especially Chapter IV of the latter, from which it takes its title, that the present essay is primarily concerned.

Before turning to the detailed examination, however, I want to offer some further general remarks about the problem, and to describe the argument in the main body of the essay. I shall begin with a brief account of the notion of sense-data and its rôle in the epistemological positions of such contemporary philosophers as Mr. Bertrand Russell, Professor Broad, and Professor G. E. Moore. Following this I shall present some preliminary observations concerning the fundamental semantic mistakes which underlie Dr. Broad's attack upon our commonplace modes of expressing perceptual judgments. The *Introduction* will conclude with a few words in explanation of my procedure and a brief synopsis of each of the six chapters to come.

THE NOTION OF SENSE-DATA

The term 'sense-data' was apparently coined by Mr. Bertrand Russell in 1912 when he wrote:

[1] The Tarner Lectures delivered in Trinity College, Cambridge, 1923.

INTRODUCTION

Let us give the name of 'sense-data' to the things that are immediately known in sensation: such things as colours, sounds, smells, hardnesses, roughnesses, and so on. We shall give the name 'sensation' to the experience of being immediately aware of these things. Thus, whenever we see a colour, we have a sensation *of* the colour, but the colour itself is a sense-datum, not a sensation. The colour is that *of* which we are immediately aware, and the awareness itself is the sensation. It is plain that if we are to know anything about the table, it must be by means of the sense-data—brown colour, oblong shape, smoothness, etc.—which we associate with the table. . . .[1]

But although the *term* 'sense-data' may be of twentieth-century coinage, the use of the notion itself, in one form or another, in epistemological analysis, is, to be sure, of respectable antiquity. As Professor Price has remarked:

. . . all past theories [of perception] have in fact started with sense-data. The Ancients and the Schoolmen called them *sensible species*. Locke and Berkeley called them *ideas of sensation*, Hume *impressions*, Kant *Vorstellungen*. In the nineteenth century they were usually known as *sensations*, and people spoke of visual and auditory sensations when they meant colour-patches and noises; while many contemporary writers, following Dr. C. D. Broad, have preferred to call them *sensa*.[2]

The notion of sense-data is, supposedly, a 'neutral' one. According to Professor Price: 'The term is meant to stand for something whose existence is indubitable (however fleeting), something from which all theories of perception ought to start, however much they may diverge later.'[3] Expressed in terms of this notion, the respects in which theories of perception may diverge concern the *nature* of sense-data, and their relation to the external physical objects of common sense. Thus, for example, the common-sense or 'naïve realist' position might be described as the theory that sense-data (excluding, of course, those which are hallucinatory or otherwise 'internal' in origin, e.g., toothache) are literally identical, both numerically and descriptively, with particular external physical objects. And the view common to the British empiricists of the seventeenth and eighteenth centuries would be that all sense-data, however they might be held to arise, and whatever they might be held to reveal about an 'external reality', are merely our own 'private mental states'.

---

1 *The Problems of Philosophy*, p. 17.
2 H. H. Price, *Perception* (1933), p. 19   3 *Loc. cit.*

3

INTRODUCTION

The character of contemporary sense-datum analysis is generally acknowledged to stem from Professor G. E. Moore's historic essay, 'The Refutation of Idealism', published in *Mind* in 1903. In this essay Professor Moore analysed sensation into two distinct elements: 'awareness', and its '*object*'; and he advanced arguments in defence of the independent existence of the latter which, with Mr. Russell, he subsequently came to call the 'sense-datum'. The effect of Professor Moore's analysis and argument was to stimulate new hope and interest in the possibility of a philosophically satisfactory empirical account of our knowledge of the external world, in terms of 'objective' sense-data.

There is, however, a vast gulf between sense-data conceived as 'colours, sounds, smells, hardnesses, roughness, and so on', and the familiar 'public' physical objects of common sense. While Professor Moore had argued, as against the views of Locke, Berkeley, Hume, and subsequent metaphysical idealists, that sense-data are not 'mental', considerations of exactly the same sort that had caused Locke to describe 'secondary qualities' as 'subjective', and which Berkeley had shown to apply to 'primary qualities' as well, still remained to challenge the identification of sense-data with physical objects as commonly conceived. If the latter are conceived to have definite shapes, sizes, colours, etc., it is argued, how are the discrepant sense-data of various individuals under different conditions to be reconciled with each other and with the external 'public' objects which they are supposed to reveal? How, for example, are the apparent ellipticity and small size of the sense-datum which one observer perceives when he views a penny obliquely and from a distance, to be reconciled with the apparent circularity and larger size of the sense-datum which another observer simultaneously perceives when he views the penny head-on and close-up; and how could both sense-data simultaneously be identified with the one penny with its one set of definite properties? And what of after-images, double vision, astigmatism, jaundice, colour-blindness, and other types of illusory and hallucinatory experience—what is the nature of the sense-data perceived in such cases, and what, if any, are the grounds for supposing such sense-data to be different from those perceived in what are called veridical cases of perception?

With these considerations in mind, many of the contemporary sense-datum analysts, such as, notably, Mr. Russell and Dr. Broad, have come to the conclusion that sense-data cannot be literally iden-

4

tified with even part of the surface of physical objects as commonly conceived, but must rather be a *tertium quid* which we are immediately aware of in sensation, and which in some way mediates our perceptual knowledge of physical objects.

Thus, Dr. Broad, for example, advances what he calls the 'Sensum Theory' concerning the nature of sense-data and their relation to physical objects. This theory, interestingly enough, is akin to the rejected historical 'Theory of Representative Ideas', the 'television theory' of perception advanced, for instance, by John Locke. The two are not, however, identical. Rather, Dr. Broad tells us, 'The doctrine of "representative ideas" is the traditional and highly muddled form of it.'[1] What the Sensum Theory does in fact hold in common with the traditional representationalist theory is the view that the 'objective constituents' of which we are immediately aware in perceptual experience are wholly private to each percipient, and are never, as is commonly supposed, literally external 'public' physical objects; and also the view that it is what we are *immediately* aware of which leads us to conceive of and believe in the existence of such objects. But here the two theories diverge in at least one major respect. Whereas, generally, the traditional theory held that what the mind knows in sensory experience is something 'mental', its own 'ideas of sensation', as Locke called them, which presumably cannot exist unperceived, the Sensum Theory holds that what is immediately revealed are 'sensa', which are 'transitory particular existents of a peculiar kind', neither physical nor mental, and not existentially dependent on being perceived, though private to and dependent on the body of each percipient.[2]

Our perception of physical objects, then, according to Dr. Broad, is of the following nature:

Under certain conditions I have states of mind called sensations. These sensations have objects, which are always concrete particular existents, like coloured or hot patches, noises, smells, etc. Such objects are called sensa. Sensa have properties, such as shape, size, hardness, colour, loudness, coldness, and so on. The existence of such sensa, and their presence to our minds in sensation, lead us to judge that a physical object exists and is present to our senses. To this physical object we ascribe various properties. These properties are not in general identical with those of the sensum which is before our minds at the moment. . . .

[1] *Scientific Thought*, p. 238.
[2] *The Mind and Its Place in Nature*, p. 181.

Nevertheless, all the properties that we do ascribe to physical objects are based upon and correlated with the properties that actually characterize our sensa.[1]

Now inevitably we find Mr. Russell and Dr. Broad raising the question whether we can possibly *know* that such things as external physical objects, as commonly conceived, exist. This is of course a logical consequence of the view that all that we ever really perceive directly are sense-data (or sensa), and that these are not to be identified with physical objects. Here is again the reply of Berkeley and Hume to Locke's notion of the 'substratum'. If all that we ever really know is one sort of thing: sense-data, what reason do we have for supposing that there is any other sort of thing: physical objects? The inferential leap from sense-data to physical objects is obviously without logical justification. For in order to infer the existence of the latter from the existence of the former, we should have to know *independently* that physical objects exist and that they are evidentially related to sense-data; and this, *ex hypothesi*, is not possible. Consequently, we find Mr. Russell advocating the thesis that physical objects are merely *logical constructs* out of sense-data,[2] and Dr. Broad saying:

We shall not then attempt to *prove* the existence of a world of entities having the constitutive properties of physical objects; for if this can be done, I at any rate do not know how to do it.[3]

And again:

The notion of Physical Object cannot be abstracted from the data of sense. It is a Category and is defined by Postulates.[4]

PROFESSOR MOORE'S POSITION

Thus far I have indicated roughly how sense-datum analysis begets scepticism concerning 'our knowledge of the external world'. Not all philosophers who begin with the notion of sense-data feel compelled to this conclusion, however. A notable exception is Professor Moore.

Although he is convinced that the 'correct analysis' of perceptual judgments must proceed from the notion of sense-data, Professor Moore employs the term in a supposedly 'neutral' sense. That is, he

[1] *Scientific Thought*, p. 243.
[2] See, for example, *Mysticism and Logic*, p. 128, and pp. 155 ff.; also, *The Analysis of Mind* (1921), p. 306.
[3] *Scientific Thought*, p. 269.   [4] *The Mind and Its Place in Nature*, p. 220.

employs the term as simply a convenient designation for 'whatever is directly perceived in sensory experience', without meaning to imply by its use any theory about the nature of sense-data or their relation to physical objects. Thus, while Dr. Broad considers it merely 'highly plausible' that there are *sensa*,[1] Professor Moore holds that it is certain that there are *sense-data*. According to him: 'The point may be put roughly by saying that what I call "sense-data" are "sensa" in Dr. Broad's sense only if the Sensum Theory is true.'[2]

The interesting thing about Professor Moore's position, however, is that in the face of the great temptation which this type of analysis offers, to which Mr. Russell and Dr. Broad, for example, have yielded, he continues steadfastly to insist upon the certainty of our common-sense knowledge about the external world of physical objects and their characteristics. Thus, in his celebrated essay 'A Defence of Common Sense',[3] he enumerates at the outset a series of commonplace propositions having to do with the existence, characteristics, and relations of familiar material things, and with our perception of them, which, as he says, some philosophers have seen fit to challenge. And he insists that not only are these commonplace propositions, and innumerable others like them, true, but that these same philosophers, no less than plain men, have *known* them to be true. Moreover, he is careful to point out that in enunciating these commonplace propositions he was not engaging in any subtle equivocation, but meant by each only its ordinary or popular meaning.

The strange thing, says Professor Moore, is that philosophers should have been able to hold sincerely, as part of their philosophical creed, propositions inconsistent with what they themselves *knew* to be true. And the source of this error, he believes, is that they have confused two quite different sets of questions. The proper questions, he insists, are not whether such commonplace propositions about material objects and our perception of them are ever true—for they certainly are, frequently—nor whether we can ever know that they are—for it is certain we can, and very often do—but rather, *how* do we know, and what is the proper *analysis* of what we know in knowing these propositions.

Now while he emphasizes that he is very doubtful, with respect to certain very important points, as to the 'correct analysis' of

---

1 Cf. *Scientific Thought*, p. 240.

2 'The Nature of Sensible Appearances', *Proc. Aristotelian Soc., Suppl. Vol. VI* (1926), pp. 183 f.

3 *Contemporary British Philosophy*, Second Series (1925), pp. 193–223.

commonplace propositions about material objects and our perception of them, Professor Moore also says that some things about this seem to him to be quite evident. And among these are that our knowledge that 'material things exist' derives from our knowledge that we do, from time to time, perceive such things as a human hand, a pen, a sheet of paper, etc.; and that our knowledge of propositions of the latter sort is deduced from propositions of the still simpler form: 'I am perceiving *this*', and, e.g., '*This* is a human hand'. Concerning the 'correct analysis' of propositions of this last form, however, he states that he is convinced only that when one knows or judges such propositions to be true,

(1) there is always some *sense-datum* about which the proposition in question is a proposition—some sense-datum which is *a* subject (and, in a certain sense, the principal or ultimate subject) of the proposition in question, and (2) that, nevertheless, *what* I am knowing or judging to be true about this sense-datum is not (in general) that it is *itself* a hand, or a dog, or the sun, etc., etc., as the case may be.[1]

In stating that sense-datum cannot be literally identified as a hand, or etc., as the case may be, Professor Moore, it should be noted, does not mean here to commit himself to the view that sense-data are sensa in Dr. Broad's sense, nor, in fact, to any view. His point is simply that any given sense-datum, if it is to be identified with a material object *at all*, can *at most* be identified only as *part of the surface of* one, since we do not see the far surface and the interior of a material object at the same time that we see its near surface. The question remains for him, then: What, precisely, *is* one knowing about the sense-datum when one knows such a proposition as 'This is a human hand'; what, precisely, *is* the relation between the sense-datum and a human hand?

It is concerning the answer to this question that Professor Moore confesses to being extremely doubtful. And this brings me to the point of this discussion of his position. As I noted at the outset, Professor Moore, while employing the sense-datum approach to the analysis of our perceptual knowledge of the external world, disavows the sceptical conclusions to which Mr. Russell and Dr. Broad have been led by it. It must not be supposed, however, that he has employed the method with impunity. For, as I want now to show, he has been able to escape the Scylla of Scepticism only by embracing the Charybdis of Paradox.

[1] *Idem*, p. 217.

INTRODUCTION

There are, Professor Moore believes, only three alternative types of answer possible to the question of the relation in perception between sense-data and material objects. One is that sense-data *themselves* are literally parts of the surfaces of particular material objects. (This would be the common-sense or 'naïve realist' view expressed in the terminology of sense-data.) Another is that sense-data are not themselves parts of the surfaces of material objects, but are only related in some more or less *'representative'* way to them. (Dr. Broad's Sensum Theory would be one form which such an answer might take.) And the third type of answer (favoured by Mr. Russell in some of his writings) is one which Professor Moore says is suggested by J. S. Mill's doctrine that material things are 'permanent possibilities of sensation'—to wit:

... that when I know such a fact as 'This is part of the surface of a human hand', what I am knowing with regard to the sense-datum which is the principal subject of that fact, is not that it is itself part of the surface of a human hand, nor yet, with regard to any relation, that *the* thing which has to it that relation is part of the surface of a human hand, but a whole set of hypothetical facts, each of which is a fact of the form 'If *these* conditions had been fulfilled, I should have been perceiving a sense-datum intrinsically related to *this* sense-datum in *this* way.' 'If *these* (other) conditions had been fulfilled, I should have been perceiving a sense-datum intrinsically related to *this* sense-datum in *this* (other) way', etc., etc.[1]

Now with respect to the latter two types of answer, it seems clear that the truth of either of them would, logically, render either uncertain or false all those commonplace propositions about material objects and our perception of them that Professor Moore stated at the outset we '*know* with certainty' to be true. For if the second type of view were correct, and all we could ever see 'directly' were sense-data, it would obviously be logically impossible for us to *know* that there were such things as particular external material objects, or that they have the particular sizes, shapes, colours, etc., which we attribute to them. While the third type of view, which denies outright that there are such things as material objects apart from 'collections of sense-data', or at least, like the second, places them beyond our ken, is in either case also clearly incompatible with the certainty of our common-sense beliefs about an external world of particular material objects having the familiar properties we associate with them.

[1] *Idem*, pp. 221 f.

9

INTRODUCTION

In view of his categorical insistence that our commonplace statements about material objects and our perception of them express, in their ordinary or popular meaning, propositions which are and which we '*know* with certainty' to be wholly and unequivocally true, it would seem, then, that Professor Moore should have no hesitation at all in rejecting these two types of answer on the basis of their logical consequences. The strange thing, however, is that while he acknowledges considerations of the sort I have noted to be 'very grave difficulties' in the way of accepting either of these two types of answer, he nevertheless says with respect to each of them, in turn, as well as with respect to the view that sense-data are literally identical with parts of the surfaces of material objects, that it 'may just possibly be the true one'.

Thus, the sense-datum approach leads, in the case of Professor Moore, admittedly not to scepticism, but yet to paradox. We '*know* with certainty' that 'material objects exist'. Our knowledge of this derives from our certain knowledge that we do, from time to time, perceive such things as a human hand, a pen, a sheet of paper, etc.; while our knowledge of the latter sort is a deduction from propositions of the still simpler form, 'I am perceiving *this*', and, e.g., '*This* is a human hand'. None the less, it may be that when we know such a proposition as '*This* is a human hand', we are knowing, about whatever it is we 'directly perceive', not that it is itself a human hand, nor even that it is part of the surface of one, but only that it is in some way 'representative' of something which is—even though, if this were the situation, it does not seem possible that we *could* know that there was such a thing, or what its particular properties were. Or again, more paradoxically still, it may be that what we are knowing, about what we 'directly perceive', is not even that it is related in any way to anything which could properly be called a human hand.

Professor Moore is not unaware, to be sure, of the paradoxes in his position. Thus, with charming and characteristic frankness, he writes:

I am now seeing part of the surface of my hand; and I do now not only feel sure but know, with regard to this object I am seeing which *is* part of the surface of my hand, *that* it is part of the surface of my hand. And also I do *now*, at the very same time, feel some doubt as to whether a certain object, which I am *directly seeing*, is identical with the object which I am seeing which is part of the surface of my hand. But to say that I feel doubt as to this, is to say that it is *possible* that it *is* identical. And, *if* it is identical, then I am both feeling sure of and doubting the very same proposition at the same time. I do not say, of course, that I *am* doing this. I only say that, so far as I can see, I don't *know* that I'm not. But it may well be thought that to say the latter is as bad as to say the former. Both are paradoxes; and there is reason to suspect that there must be something wrong in the premisses which lead me to say the latter. Yet I cannot see what *is* wrong with them, if anything is. Perhaps the most fundamental puzzle about the relation of sense-data to physical objects is that there does seem to be reason to assert the latter of these two paradoxes.[1]

What it is that persuades so careful a philosopher as Professor Moore to entertain such absurd paradoxes seriously—rather than to conclude simply that since our indubitable knowledge that 'material objects exist' and that they have the characteristics they sensibly appear to us to have would be logically impossible on any other formula, we *must* perceive external material objects 'directly'—is, of course, that he is unable to get over the same stumbling block that has led Mr. Russell and Dr. Broad, among others, to scepticism. How are the discrepant sense-data of various individuals under different conditions to be reconciled with each other and with the external 'public' objects which they are supposed to reveal? This, in all its variations, is the problem that has troubled contemporary sense-datum analysts ever since the turn of the century, and, in one form or another, their philosophical ancestors before them. Strangely enough, however, they never consider the possibility that the sense-datum approach itself may be at fault.

Now there are, to be sure, cases in which people are mistaken in supposing themselves to be perceiving a material object at all, let alone a material surface of a particular kind—e.g., after-images, dreams, hallucinations. And such perceptual experiences do resemble those which are veridical, and may even sometimes, taken by themselves, be indistinguishable from them. And there are also various types of illusions in which, under certain conditions, physical objects may appear to have properties they do not have, or may appear not to have properties they do have. Because of such situations and the mistaken judgments to which they sometimes give rise, some philosophers think it justified in epistemological analysis to regard *every* perceptual judgment, whether or not the perception from which it stems is, in the ordinary sense, veridical, as a judgment

[1] 'A Reply to My Critics', *The Philosophy of G. E. Moore*, Library of Living Philosophers (1942), p. 637.

not about a material object, nor even about part of the surface of one, but rather about the percipient's own, in some sense 'private', '*sense-datum*'.

We are asked to believe that the term 'sense-datum' is a '*neutral*' term, standing for something whose existence is indubitable, with the door left open for it to be identified, if there is warrant, with the surface of a particular material object. Now if the term 'sense-datum' were consistently regarded only as an intentionally ambiguous term which could be used to refer, alternatively, to part of the surface of a material object in cases of veridical perception, and to an 'hallucinatory image' in cases of this type, the procedure might be innocent enough. But it seem inevitable that those who employ this type of approach to the analysis of our perceptual knowledge of the external world should fall victim to certain forms of expression, and consequently, to certain ways of thinking, in which the 'sense-datum' is hypostatized into a kind of filmy thing having existence and properties in its own right—a *tertium quid* mediating between perceiver and external world. Thus, from this allegedly 'neutral' beginning, we find such philosophers as Dr. Broad and Mr. Russell concluding that we cannot *know* that there is an external world of material objects, and that, if there is, its nature must be quite different from what it is commonly conceived to be. And we find Professor Moore puzzling with them as to how the 'sense-datum' which we 'directly see' when we look obliquely at a penny can be identical with the face of the penny, since the latter is circular, while the sense-datum '*is*' elliptical; and hence, despite his conviction that we certainly *do* know, puzzling as to *how*, exactly, we know that there are material objects and that they have the properties we associate with them—as though it were not enough to say that we know because we see them and feel them, and not enough to cite the well-known facts of physiology, psychology, and optics.

When I come in the succeeding chapters to discuss Dr. Broad's arguments in detail, I shall try to show that this analytic procedure is not justified by the existence of either hallucinatory or illusory perception. And I shall also try to make clear just how the sense-datum approach, far from being epistemologically neutral, separates perceiver and 'external world' from the start by a logically impenetrable veil.

INTRODUCTION

PROFESSOR BROAD AND ORDINARY LANGUAGE

In the preceding section I indicated how Professor Moore's predilection for sense-datum analysis leads him to paradox rather than to scepticism concerning 'our knowledge of the external world'. Whether or not his conception of analysis is incompatible with his defence of common sense, he is certainly correct, I am convinced, in his uncompromising insistence that our commonplace modes of expression about material objects and our perception of them can and do very often, in their ordinary or popular meaning, express propositions which are wholly and unequivocally true, and which, moreover, we can and do very often *know* to be true. And I want now to contrast this view with Dr. Broad's.

As Mr. John Wisdom has remarked:

... though Broad sometimes speaks, like Moore, as if philosophy were the job of finding the analysis of what is naturally indicated by phrases like 'I am seeing a chair', 'I am hearing a bell', he more often speaks of it as if it were the finding of the most probable hypothesis explanatory of what we can in the strictest sense observe—as if it were science, only more so ... as though it were a matter of finding out how much is probably true of what we ordinarily mean by such statements as 'The earth has existed for many years past', 'I have half a crown left'. He often speaks as if, although these statements in so far as they merely record and predict the observable are unquestionable, they are nevertheless questionable in respect of a hypothesis tacitly assumed in them.[1]

Thus, for example, Dr. Broad begins his argument in Chapter IV of *The Mind and Its Place in Nature* with the innocent enough statement that no one doubts that such phrases as 'I see a bell', 'I feel a bell', 'I hear a bell' indicate 'states of affairs which actually exist from time to time', and that—what is likewise true enough, among philosophers—'People do not begin to quarrel till they try to *analyse* such situations. . . .' This would appear to be quite compatible with Professor Moore's position. Immediately, however, he goes on to say:

When they do this they are liable to find that the only senses of 'I', 'bell', and 'hear', which will make the statement true are very different from those which we are wont to attach to those words. If this should happen, it still remains true, of course, that the phrases 'I hear a bell'

1 'Moore's Technique', in *The Philosophy of G. E. Moore*, P. A. Schilpp, ed. (1942), p. 427.

and 'I see a chair' stand for real states of affairs which differ in certain specific ways from each other; but these states of affairs may be extremely different in their structure and their components from what the form of words used to indicate them would naturally suggest to us.[1]

And this seems to be precisely the sort of view which Professor Moore meant to disavow when he wrote, concerning the set of commonplace indubitable propositions which he enumerates in his 'A Defence of Common Sense':

> Some philosophers seem to have thought it legitimate to use such expressions . . . as if they expressed something which they really believed, when in fact they believe that every proposition, which such an expression would *ordinarily* be understood to express, is, at least partially, false; and all they really believe is that there is some *other* set of propositions, related in a certain way to those which such expressions do actually express, which, unlike these, really are true. . . . I wish, therefore, to make it quite plain that I was not using the expressions . . . in any such subtle sense. I meant by each of them precisely what every reader, in reading them, will have understood me to mean. And any philosopher, therefore, who holds that any of these expressions, if understood in this popular manner, expresses a proposition which embodies some popular error, is disagreeing with me. . . .[2]

At the bottom of Dr. Broad's reservations concerning our commonplace modes of expression is what he terms the 'Principle of Exceptional Cases'.[3] 'If we want to clear up the meaning of some commonly used concept', he states, 'it is enormously important to see how it applies to exceptional cases.' Thus, for instance, he proposes to 'clarify' the concept 'being in a place' in such a way that it will answer equally well the question 'Where is the mirror-image of a pin?' and the question 'Where is the pin itself?' In theory, he says, one either could take the sense in which the pin itself is in its place as fundamental, and try to 'explain' the sense in which the image is in *its* place 'by making a number of supplementary hypotheses'; or else one could take the sense in which the image is in its place as fundamental, and regard the facts which are true of the pin and not of the image, as due to the fulfilment of certain special conditions, which need not be realized, but which in fact generally are. The latter, he says, 'seems to be the only hopeful course to take'.

[1] Pp. 140 f.   [2] *Loc. cit.*, pp. 197 f.
[3] 'Critical and Speculative Philosophy', *Contemporary British Philosophy*, First Series (1924), pp. 90 f.

INTRODUCTION

Ordinary usage, Dr. Broad maintains, reflects popular, common-sense beliefs about the world and our perception of it which we have uncritically inherited from our practical-minded prehistoric ancestors; and these beliefs will not stand up when we take into account all the factors which were ignored in their development. It is natural, he says, that when we do consider these factors we find the beliefs far too simple-minded to deal with the extremely complex situation. And thus he argues that what is required if our ordinary statements are to fit the facts is a re-definition of such commonplace terms as 'I', 'see', 'physical object', 'place', etc.

Now if Dr. Broad's aim were merely that of linguistic reform, his desire for generality would be purely a matter of personal taste. And though the magnitude and complexity of the task is exhausting even to contemplate, there is in theory, so far as I can see, no reason why it would not be possible, given enough patience, time, and ingenuity, to construct a calculus of words in which everything that one might wish to say in ordinary language could be rendered, but in which the vocabulary and the rules governing the formation, transformation, and combination of expressions would be precisely and consistently defined and formulated. Thus, to suggest one small area of possible labour, such words and phrases as 'in my' and 'I have' would either need to be restricted in their use, or else re-defined in such a way that they would have a common meaning in such different contexts as 'in my pocket', 'in my mind', 'in my position'; 'I have a desk', 'I have a hand', 'I have a toothache', etc., etc.

But clearly Dr. Broad is not advocating linguistic reconstruction for its own sake. Rather, to pursue Mr. Wisdom's suggestion in the quotation above, Dr. Broad's remarks are more reminiscent of the scientist. Thus, like the scientist, who is concerned to reduce the 'explanation' of natural phenomena to the smallest possible number of primitive concepts and laws, Dr. Broad wishes, for example, to fit the phenomena of a pin and its mirror-image to a single concept of 'being in a place'. And again, just as the scientist aims at an exact and elegant language in which every term is precisely defined and in which all syntactical rules are explicitly and consistently formulated, so Dr. Broad desires a re-definition of commonplace terms and expressions so that they might have a consistent meaning in all cases, abnormal as well as normal.

The question is, however, supposing that the kind of linguistic reconstruction that Dr. Broad has in mind were accomplished, what would it profit us? Would it, like the language of the physicist or the chemist, for example, enable us to deal quantitatively with complex, interrelated phenomena, and thus to discover previously hidden functional relationships, or previously unknown entities or processes? Would it enable us to predict and control the order of events in the empirical world in a way not possible or feasible with ordinary language and the languages of mathematics and the natural sciences? I do not think so, and I do not believe that Dr. Broad does either.

What, then, is the explanation of the importance which he attaches to linguistic reconstruction? It is to be found, I think, in his conviction that we are forever shut up behind the impenetrable curtain of our 'sense-data' and can at best only infer or surmise, from our 'immediate awareness' of them, the nature of the 'external world' beyond. Obviously it would matter little what particular notational system were employed to deal with *entirely observable* situations, so long as we could in pragmatically successful fashion record, predict, and communicate about the observable relationships, patterns, sequences, characteristics, and the like. All that would be required is a conventional vocabulary and syntax sufficiently detailed and articulated to represent whatever could be perceived. To wish to reconstruct such a language, it is clear, would be no more than a desire for linguistic nicety. For since the terms and syntax of the language would represent only the observable kinds of situations for which the language was designed, and would do so by arbitrary convention, there could be no such thing as a fundamental misrepresentation implicit in the vocabulary and structure of the language itself. There could, of course, in the ordinary sense, be false statements about the observable; and there could be linguistic misuse, or violations of the established notational conventions. But when an expression was being used to represent the kind of situation in terms of which it had been ostensively defined—i.e., in the presence of which its first users had adopted and its subsequent users had been taught the convention for its use—there would be no sense to the charge that it did not represent that kind of situation properly. Thus, if that type of totally observable situation were at any time the case, the expression in indicating it would at that time, or with respect to that time, express a proposition which was wholly and unequivocally true.

In suggesting, then, that the ordinary modes of expression in which we describe the perceptual situations 'I see a chair', 'I hear a bell', etc., might not *ever*, in their ordinary sense, accurately represent what is actually the case when such situations exist, it is clear that Dr. Broad must have in mind some distinction between 'appearance' and 'reality'. The kind of situation he must have in mind is something like the following, reminiscent of Plato's 'Allegory of the Cave' in the seventh book of *The Republic*. Suppose we were watching a shadow-play on a translucent screen. The light source is behind the screen, and the objects causing the shadows to appear on the screen are between it and the light source, hidden from our direct view. With the circumstances thus, the shadows which could be caused to appear on the screen in the form of persons, animals, and various familiar objects, in various familiar motions and relationships, might very well be produced by quite different objects in quite different motions and relations. In describing in ordinary language the appearances on the screen, however, we would quite naturally speak in terms of the real objects and relations which the shadows were supposed to represent. And thus our expressions, despite their practical usefulness for describing the observable shadow-world, would not, or at least might not, represent accurately the constituents and relations of the actual situation behind the screen.

Now, since Dr. Broad is convinced that the 'external world' is hidden from us by the mediating sense-data which *are* supposed to be 'directly revealed' in perception, he similarly conceives it to be entirely possible that the 'ultimate' things and relations in the 'external world' should be quite different from the things and relations which we uncritically take our sense-data to reveal. Thus, while he says that there is no doubt that such expressions as 'I see a bell', 'I feel a bell', 'I hear a bell', stand for real states of affairs which actually exist from time to time and which differ in certain specific ways from each other, he also says that these states of affairs may be extremely different in their structure and their components from what the form of words used to indicate them would naturally suggest. In other words, while the ordinary modes of expression may serve well enough to indicate the observable patterns and sequences of events on our curtain of sense-data, so to speak, they may not be at all accurate as a description of what must ultimately be the case.

Unlike the situation of observing the shadow-play on the screen, however, it is not possible to escape the screen of sense-data and perceive directly what, if anything, lies beyond. Thus, what is necessary is by the *analysis* of the patterns and sequences of sense-data of which we are directly aware in perception, to try to arrive at a coherent and consistent *theory* concerning the nature of sense-data, their relation to the supposed external world, and the nature of this world. And the result of this enterprise will naturally determine the proper form which the perceptual judgments we express must take if they are to render the actual situation accurately.

The question, therefore, is whether or not the situation with respect to *ordinary* perception and our customary modes of representing it is, as Dr. Broad conceives it to be, like the situation of the shadow-play described above. Now in the chapters to follow I shall try to show that it is the sense-datum approach itself that begets the difficulties which Dr. Broad finds in the 'common-sense view' concerning our perceptual knowledge of physical objects, and that leads him to this misconception. But here I want to call attention to some basic linguistic considerations which underlie my argument in those chapters, and which, I think, show the initial absurdity of the suggestion that such an expression as 'I see a chair' might intrinsically misrepresent the situations in which it is customarily employed.

Several paragraphs above I suggested that to wish to reconstruct a notational system that had been devised to deal with wholly observable situations could be no more than a desire for neatness and elegance. For the meaning of the expressions in such a language would be established ostensively, in the presence of just those kinds of situation thereafter to be understood as denoted by them; and there could thus be no question of misrepresentation. The expressions in such a language would not *predicate* anything about the situations with respect to which they were employed, but would merely *designate* them, by arbitrary convention. Or, to put the point another way, what they would predicate with respect to these situations would be only their immediately or ultimately perceptible similarity, in essential features, to the original ostensive defining situations.

Now it must be seen that what is true of the hypothetical language about which I have been speaking is true of *any* natural language; for instance, ordinary English. And especially is it true of the ordinary, common-sense modes of expression in which we express our perceptual judgments about physical objects. After all, we do not think and speak in words from birth, but must *learn* language. And we cannot learn it by being shown a list of words and rules of grammatical syntax, or by hearing such a list pronounced; nor, obviously, can we be taught it initially by verbal explanation. To perceive a word or an expression at this stage is to perceive a mere sequence of sounds or marks. A picture 'carries its meaning' with it, so to speak; but the non-imitative, arbitrary sounds or marks, which are the words and phrases of ordinary language, clearly do not. Given an egg in the shell, a child may, without help or the opportunity for observation and imitation, chance to break open the shell and discover by himself the egg inside; but he obviously couldn't discover the meaning of words and sentences in this way. For their meaning is *given* to them.

Words and sentences 'mean' because *we* mean. That is, their meaning is a matter of their use or function, not an intrinsic property. To give meaning to a word or sentence is to specify the convention for its use or application. And with respect to the basic terms and expressions of a natural language, this is and can only be accomplished by using them in the presence of the kinds of perceptible things, qualities, relations, and the like, which are to be understood by them. Thus, as children, we are taught the conventional meaning of the sounds and marks in an already established language by witnessing their use in appropriate situations; and whether or not we have learned the convention for their use —i.e., their 'meaning'—is demonstrated by our using them in such observably appropriate circumstances and not in inappropriate ones. And of course the same process held for our teachers when *they* learned to use these words and phrases in *their* childhood, and for their teachers before them. And so on back to the beginnings of language, when those prehistoric ancestors to whom Dr. Broad refers first began to use sounds and marks to represent common experience.

With these considerations in mind, then, the initial absurdity of Dr. Broad's suggestion that analysis may reveal that our commonplace modes of expressing perceptual judgments actually misrepresent the situations they are employed to designate should be clear. These modes of expression cannot misrepresent the ordinary situations in which they are customarily employed; for they were ostensively defined in terms of just such situations, and they mean nothing more than what is sensibly revealed in them. When we say, for example, in the ordinary situation, 'I see a tree', this expression is intended to convey only the kind of commonplace observable situation in terms of which we were taught its use or meaning. Having from childhood on experienced this kind of situation, and having learned that it is the kind of situation which the sound or mark 'I see a tree' is customarily used to represent, we in turn employ it whenever we wish to indicate that type of situation. In short, whenever we express a perceptual judgment in terms of one of these commonplace expressions, all that the use of that particular expression signifies is that we are judging the situation in question to be, in the relevant observable respects, like the innumerable previously experienced situations in which we learned and exercised the conventions governing its use.[1] And if the situation to which we apply it is indeed like those in which we were taught its use, there can be no question of misrepresentation.

Dr. Broad's statement that we have inherited our commonplace modes of expression from our prehistoric ancestors may very well be true. But just as it would be palpably senseless to suggest that those who first employed some arbitrary sound, such as 'green', or its prehistoric equivalent, to stand for the perceptibly distinguishable colour of, say, the leaves on the trees in summer, may have been mistaken in employing that otherwise meaningless sound rather than another, so there is also no sense in the suggestion that our prehistoric ancestors could somehow have been mistaken when they first employed such an expression as 'I see a tree', or whatever comparable expression they did employ—as though the expression really had some innate or prior meaning, or as though the situation which it was arbitrarily used to designate had its own proper designation, quite apart from any that might be humanly devised for it.

Dr. Broad thinks that our commonplace modes of expressing perceptual judgments might be mistaken because he conceives them to express *hypotheses* about perceptual data. In taking issue with what he terms 'the common-sense view', he does not deny, as I have noted, that such 'states of affairs' as are 'naturally indicated' by commonplace expressions like 'I see a chair', 'I see a bell', 'I hear a bell', etc., actually exist from time to time; nor does he deny that these everyday expressions adequately serve to denote and distinguish these different 'perceptual situations' for purely practical purposes. But he has in mind a certain 'uncritical

1 In this sense aren't *all* assertive judgments ultimately *judgments of comparison*?

belief', or '*a priori* assumption', which he supposes to be reflected in the very form of all such expressions, and to be implicit in the particular perceptual judgments we express by means of them—a belief or assumption respecting an 'external world' lying forever beyond, as he claims to show, what can in the strictest sense be observed. Specifically, he identifies as 'the common-sense view' the general 'belief' that 'Physical objects, literally extended in space and time, and having all the qualities and properties we commonly attribute to them, exist, and are "directly revealed" in sense-perception.' And it is in so far as they involve a commitment to this 'belief' that he holds that our particular common-sense perceptual judgments must be construed as hypotheses about perceptual data.

Now to begin with, it should be clear from the argument of the preceding paragraphs that the forms of expression we employ in everyday, common-sense discourse about our perceptual experience do not involve an uncritical belief or *a priori* commitment about anything whatsoever, let alone about a supposed 'ultimately unknowable external world'. For as I have tried to show, they merely comprise a naturally evolved, more or less coherent system of notational conventions for representing the recurrent kinds and patterns of entities, relations, qualities and properties which we first discern and then come to expect in sense-perception.

To be sure, it may be held that all such expressions, in so far as they purport to refer to a situation involving, e.g., an actual tree, and not merely an ingeniously contrived artificial one, or a two-dimensional representation of a tree, and in so far also as they purport to describe actual perceptions and not mere hallucinations, *do* imply something beyond the *immediately* observable about the situations to which they are applied. Or again, it may be held that such a judgment as 'I see a *metal* chair' asserts something which cannot, at least always, be ascertained by simple visual inspection. But such 'hypotheses', of course, are ultimately decidable by further or more careful observation, or by application of the proper definitional tests.

In suggesting that the general statement which he identifies as 'the common-sense view' is merely an hypothesis about perceptual data, and that particular judgments such as 'I see a chair' must be mistaken or at least doubtful in so far as they entail this general statement, Dr. Broad has a quite different kind of 'hypothesis' in mind, however; one which could not possibly be decided within perceptual experience. For what he is suggesting is not that our commonplace perceptual judgments are hypotheses in so far as they relate particular items of perceptual experience to further possible experience, but rather that they are hypotheses about perceptual data *as a whole*—i.e., hypotheses referring, so to speak, *'beyond'* the totality of whatever is or ever could be revealed in experience.

But how could our commonplace expressions possibly represent such 'hypotheses'? The point should be borne in mind that in itself any assertive expression is, after all, only a sequence of arbitrary marks or sounds, its meaning accruing to it solely by convention. Hence, for such expressions to signify anything to us, we must be party to the convention governing their use. That is, we must be acquainted with the state of affairs, or at least the *kind* of state of affairs, which each given form of expression is to be understood to symbolize, so that whenever that expression is used in subsequent assertion we may understand just what is being claimed to be the case. And ultimately, as I have said, we must learn the convention for the use of arbitrary symbols by literally observing their use in appropriate circumstances. For the alternative, verbal definition, can function, of course, only if we have already learned the meaning of the defining words and phrases, and so provides no ultimate escape from the necessity of ostensive definition. This being appreciated, the absurdity of Dr. Broad's suggestion should be apparent. How could our commonplace expressions about physical objects and perceptions—or *any* expression, for that matter—possibly acquire for us the alleged 'trans-experiential' meaning which he supposes them to have in addition to what they mean in terms of possible sense-experience? How, for instance, could anyone learn or teach another this additional meaning supposed to be conveyed by such an expression as 'I see a tree', if neither it nor even the alleged additional meaning for any other expression of its type had ever been or could ever be perceptibly exemplified? And what is more, how could we possibly have come to understand the very words Dr. Broad employs in explaining to us just what implications of these assertive expressions he wishes to question? Obviously, for Dr. Broad to be correct in his contention that our commonplace expressions refer 'beyond' possible experience, we would be obliged to assume that we could know at least part of their meaning *a priori*, even though they are supposed to express entirely contingent propositions. And this is patently absurd.

Statements of the general type: 'Physical objects exist', 'Physical objects have shape, size, qualities, etc.', and 'Physical objects are "directly revealed" in perception', which Dr. Broad takes to be hypotheses about perceptual data implied by our commonplace modes of expression, are not factual assertions in their own right, it should be recognized. They are merely shorthand expressions, as it were, abstract generalizations of a peculiar sort, reflecting the form of the countless *particular* assertions we make about the existence and specific characteristics of the particular objects and kinds of objects (tables, chairs, trees, books) which we encounter in sense-perception, and about the conditions under which we perceive them. Expressions of the general type bear much the same relation, logically, to the particular expressions, that a statement of the form 'This object is coloured' bears to a statement like 'This object is red'. If the particular statements are true, then the general statements are also true, by definition; while the particular statements are true whenever the appropriate circumstances are realized. And since the expressions in which we formulate the particular assertions are, after all, arbitrary and conventional, and hence can signify no more than what is revealed in the particular perceptual situations or sequences of perceptual situations in terms of which they must be defined, it follows that the general statements cannot signify anything more, either.

Dr. Broad's reference to 'the *analyses* made unconsciously for practical ends by our prehistoric ancestors', which our commonplace modes of expression are supposed to reflect, can likewise be shown to be a semantic muddle.

The modes of expression which we have inherited from our prehistoric ancestors inevitably suggest a certain mode of analysis for the situations to which they are applied, he tells us. The expression 'I see a chair' suggests that the perceptual situation thus indicated 'consists of me and the physical object whose name appears in the phrase, related directly by an asymmetrical two-term relation which is indicated by the verb'. And while it is 'plausible' to suppose that the situation does contain two outstanding constituents related in this way, he says, 'it is quite another question whether these two constituents can possibly be what is commonly understood by "me" and by "chair"'.

Now, in the first place, to suggest even the bare possibility that the type of situation normally indicated by the expression 'I see a chair' may not *really* 'contain two outstanding constituents', but that this merely reflects a tacit, uncritical 'analysis' made by our prehistoric ancestors, is not, I want to show, to suggest anything meaningful at all. Which of the 'constituents' of any situation are 'outstanding' is, of course, a function of interest or attention. And that the recurrent kinds and patterns of entities, relations, qualities, and properties which we distinguish in perceptual experience and designate by language all reflect a practical concern cannot be denied—any more than it can be denied, for that matter, that the subtlety of the discriminations of similarity and difference which people are accustomed to make among the data of perception determine, and are reciprocally facilitated or discouraged by, the richness or poverty of the vocabulary and syntax of their particular language. But granted that our ancestors, as we, found it natural to describe perceptual situations in terms of a perceiver and some perceived object, what is the nature of the 'analysis' which Dr. Broad says is involved? For there to be descriptive assertion at all, *some* selection from the total complex situation must be made. Recognizably recurrent aspects of experience must be distinguished, and a convention established for representing them by the otherwise meaningless, arbitrary sounds or marks which are the words and phrases of language. And it is only *after* such a notational system is established that the correctness or incorrectness of a particular *subsequent* descriptive assertion can be judged —in terms of the likeness or unlikeness, in the essential respects, of the situation in question to the defining situation or situations in which the notational convention was initially established. With respect to the initial defining situations themselves, however, no such judgment can be made; for without an antecedent standard there is simply no meaning to a judgment of correctness or incorrectness.

It would be possible, I suppose, to construct a language with terminological classifications straddling the perceptual discriminations we are accustomed to make, just as the stars in the sky comprising the various familiar constellations might have been conventionally grouped to form other visual configurations, or just as the zoölogical phyla might have been arranged quite differently if other principles of classification had been employed. And perhaps such a language would also require a correspondingly modified syntax. But what representational advantage would be gained by such linguistic alteration? To be understood by their users, the expressions in the revised language would, like the expressions of the familiar natural languages, have to be assigned their meanings at least ultimately by reference to concrete, perceptible situations. And any observable situation that could be represented in the revised language could also be represented in any other rich and sufficiently articulated language—in such a language, for instance, as ordinary English. Since, then, the revised language and the familiar natural languages would be no more than alternative modes of representing the perceptible aspects of immediately or at least ultimately observable situations, the expressions in one language could not be said to describe the 'actual situations' more accurately than the expressions in another, any more than visually selecting and grouping the stars in the sky to form constellations different from those we conventionally distinguish could be said to represent the sensible pattern of the stars more accurately.

So long as we select elements that we can distinguish in common with other persons, we can establish a linguistic convention for descriptive assertion that will be adequate for whatever situations we may observe. And it can make no sense to say that our descriptive expressions might be intrinsically inaccurate; for they have no other meaning than the distinguishable aspects of experience which they were devised to represent and which the parties to the linguistic convention understand them to represent. Thus, to suggest that the situations we normally describe by such expressions as 'I see a chair', 'I hear a bell', etc., may not really contain the two 'outstanding constituents' whose names appear in the expressions would be to suggest that we have not really discerned in these situations any such recognizably recurrent elements as we customarily and arbitrarily designate by the two terms. And this is so manifestly false that Dr. Broad clearly shies from it.

Instead he says, as I have noted, that while it is 'plausible' to suppose that the perceptual situation does contain two 'outstanding constituents', the question is whether these two constituents can possibly be what is commonly understood by 'me' and by 'chair' (or etc.). But this, it should be appreciated, will not do either. For the same arguments which applied to the suggestion that our commonplace forms of expression might misrepresent the situations they were devised to denote also apply here.

In their ordinary meaning such terms as 'I', 'see', 'chair', etc., do not designate abstract notions which we acquire by verbal explanation and about which we may hence have misconceptions. Rather we learn their meaning ostensively, by observing their use in the concrete situations of everyday life. And what is 'commonly understood' by them, therefore, is just what is distinguishably revealed in those perceptual situations, or sequences of perceptual situations, of everyday life. In the chapters to come I shall show that Dr. Broad's procedure is to define such terms in abstraction, and then to deny that expressions involving them express anything that is confirmed by experience. But obviously, any interpretation of these ostensively defined words and phrases from which it follows that they have no exemplification or that they do not accurately represent what is revealed in perceptual experience must be a misinterpretation.

To illustrate: A formal statement of the commonly understood meaning of the term 'physical object' might conceivably include some such proposition as that it stands for something which normally has a 'continuing identity' over an appreciable period of time. Suppose now it were scientifically proclaimed that the individual molecules composing macroscopic physical objects are completely replaced every one-thousandth of a second by exchange with like molecules from the surrounding environment. The newspapers might very well describe such a theoretical development as 'the astounding scientific discovery that physical objects do not, as popularly thought, have continuous identities'. But in truth such a 'discovery' would no more render untenable the commonly understood meaning of 'physical object' as involving 'continuing identity' than did the molecular theory of the composition of matter controvert what we ordinarily mean when we speak of a chair, for example, as being a 'solid object'. For if the phrase 'having a continuing identity over an appreciable period of time' is intended to represent part of the commonly understood meaning of the term 'physical object', it must be interpreted not in some theoretical or ideal sense, but in the ordinary sense; and this is the sense in which even a philosopher could identify his hat in the cloak-room and would lodge a complaint with the management if it were not there when he returned, or if it had been exchanged for another.

I want finally to say something about my method of procedure in the detailed examination of Dr. Broad's views which follows, and to describe briefly the content of each of the six chapters.

My aim in this essay, as I have indicated, is to defend the common-sense notions and expressions about our perception of physical objects against the attack of sense-datum analysis, and to show how the epistemological problems generated by this type of approach and the paradoxical conclusions to which they lead can be dissolved by due regard for the logic of ordinary language. Because the linguistically-oriented method of analysis which I employ requires careful attention to the actual wording of the views I am concerned to refute as well as to the general structure of their argument, the essay, as I have said, is limited primarily to a single formulation: the clear and concise presentation in Chapter IV, 'Sense-Perception and Matter', of Dr. Broad's *The Mind and Its Place in Nature* (1925). Occasionally I have also referred to the somewhat more detailed and expanded statement of his views which he gives in Chapter VII, 'Matter and Its Appearances,' and Chapter VIII, 'The Theory of Sensa and the Critical Scientific Theory', of his earlier work, *Scientific Thought* (1923); but the organization of my essay follows closely that of Chapter IV in the former work.

The method of procedure I have employed is to present Dr. Broad's argument in this chapter step by step and in his own words, so far as practicable, introducing critical analysis and discussion as I go along. This mode of procedure, it must be admitted, since it requires frequent recapitulation of both exposition and criticism to preserve continuity, has resulted in a certain amount of repetition that might have been avoided by a more synoptic treatment. But the thesis that the development of Dr. Broad's argument depends for its cogency in large part on an accumulation of subtle linguistic mistakes and confusions seemed to me to call for a method of analytic procedure that would permit their exposure when and as they occur. The illusive familiarity or 'transparency' of language makes it no easy task to demonstrate linguistic error convincingly by *any* method, however, and a certain amount of repetitiousness is due, not to the piecemeal procedure, but simply to the fact that in trying to put what I may judge to be a particularly subtle or important point clearly and effectively, I sometimes adopt several different approaches.

As for the critical analysis and discussion itself, it proceeds along the lines set forth in the preceding section. By appealing to everyday facts and linguistic usage, by explicating the 'logic' inherent in ordinary usage, and in large part simply by restating the facts to which he alludes, and the conclusions he draws from them, into more familiar, common-sense language, I have been able in every case, I believe, to dissipate the problems which Dr. Broad generates concerning our perceptual knowledge of physical objects, and to show that his 'solutions' are merely verbal. On the whole, Dr. Broad's admirably lucid and explicit style of presentation has facilitated the task of analysis and criticism. In some few cases, however, I have been unable to penetrate his meaning or to discover the process of reasoning which would lead him to draw the conclusions he does from the facts he adduces. In those cases I am obliged to deny him the benefit of the doubt. For, as I maintain throughout, any argument or analysis which purports to show that beliefs and expressions whose very *sense* derives from everyday, pragmatically successful usage are incorrect or inaccurate must *ipso facto*, like the paradoxical 'proofs' of Zeno, be false and sophistical.

To conclude this *Introduction*, the synopsis of the six chapters comprising the essay follows:

In *Chapter I*, 'The "Facts" of Perception', I present and discuss critically Dr. Broad's preliminary statement of the problem, and of what he considers to be the facts which 'everyone, whatever his philosophical views may be, would admit'. The development of his ensuing argument is foreshadowed and facilitated by his classification of hallucinatory experiences at the outset with veridical perceptual experiences (in contradistinction to experiences of the type: 'I feel cross') on the basis of 'the claim to external cognitive contact'. This claim he designates by saying that they both 'have epistemological objects', the difference between the two being merely the presence or absence of a corresponding 'onto-logical object'. By stating the facts thus, I argue, Dr. Broad im-plicitly introduces the ensnaring notion of the 'sense-datum' of which we are supposed to be immediately aware in both veridical and hallucinatory perceptual experience; and this leads inevitably to the logically unsolvable problem of how cognitive contact with external 'ontological objects' is possible, if all one is ever immedi-ately aware of in perceptual experience are 'epistemological ob-jects'. In this connection I also examine what Dr. Broad means by 'sensation', and his conception of its role in perception. I take issue with the supposition that one can distinguish (e.g.) a 'brown patch of such and such a shápe, etc.'—in Dr. Broad's later termin-ology, a 'sensum'— from the chair which one perceives, and also with his description of perception as an 'emergent characteristic' arising from the sensation of simple qualities.

Chapter II, ' "Physical Object" and "Objective Constituent" ', is concerned with Dr. Broad's argument that 'perceptual situa-tions' do not literally 'contain as a constituent' anything properly termed a 'physical object', and that our common-sense forms of expression represent untenable 'simple-minded analyses made unconsciously for practical ends by our prehistoric ancestors'. Anything that we should be willing to call a 'physical object', he argues, must have duration, unity, and continuity; must have an inside as well as an outside; and must have other qualities besides those immediately revealed to a particular sense. In a given per-ceptual situation, however, one is directly aware, he says, of only a 'short event which is, at most, a slice of a longer strand of history which is the history of the particular object'; furthermore, one is directly aware of only a small part of its outside near surface; and finally, one is sensuously aware of only a small selection of the total qualities it is supposed to have. Pointing out, to begin with, the strangeness of Dr. Broad's preliminary suggestion that there may not even *be* things which in fact have all the required charac-teristics (since the denotation of the term 'physical object' obvi-ously antedated its connotation, and any statement of the latter must be interpreted by reference to the former), I go on to argue that he misrepresents the common-sense belief about our percep-tion of physical objects. It does not hold, as his argument suggests, that in seeing a physical object one sees its far side and its inside at the same time or in the same sense that one sees its near surface, or etc., but only that one is seeing something which does in fact—as may be confirmed by further perception—have all the properties required for it to count as a physical object. Dr. Broad's definition of the limits of the 'perceptual situation', and his conception of the 'objective constituent' from the outset not as a physical object, but as a kind of 'sensory image', as I try to show, are arbitrary and artificial, and beg the question of whether or not physical objects are 'directly revealed' in perceptual situations.

The discussion in *Chapter III*, 'The "External Reference" of Perception', is divided into two main parts: (i) The 'External Reference', and (ii) The Relevance of Delusive Perception. By the former Dr. Broad means 'the conviction that the "given" or "objective constituent" of a single perceptual situation is part of a larger whole of a certain characteristic kind, viz., a certain physical object, and that this whole has other qualities besides those which are sensuously manifested in the perceptual situation'. Although I agree with Dr. Broad that it is a matter of psychological observation that perception does not involve *inference* from 'given objective constituents', and that the strength of the 'conviction of external reference' could not at any rate be justified thus, I maintain that he is mistaken in concluding that 'the notion of persistent physical objects is logically merely an hypothesis to explain the correlations between perceptual situations'. Of the different types of scientific hypotheses I describe, Dr. Broad's conception of the notion of external physical objects seems most akin to scientific 'explanations' of observable macroscopic interrelations in terms of postulated *constructs*—e.g., molecules, atoms, electrons—which are inaccessible to direct observation. But to characterize the notion of physical objects as a *'mere hypothesis'*, I argue, is a fundamental linguistic confusion. For it misleadingly suggests that there is something always lacking in our knowledge of physical objects, some theoretical 'more ideal' or direct kind of knowledge; whereas it is the very directness and ideality of our ordinary perceptual acquaintance with physical objects and their relations that provides the basis of comparison for distinguishing *other* notions or beliefs as *'merely'* hypothetical.

The second part of this chapter deals with Dr. Broad's contention that 'since there is no relevant internal difference between the veridical and the delusive perceptual situation, it is reasonable to suppose that in no case does a perceptual situation contain as a constituent the physical object which corresponds to its epistemological object, even when there is such a physical object'; and that, further, since the claim of 'external reference' is false in *some* cases, it cannot be accepted as true merely at its face-value in *any* case, and may be wrong in all. Here my reply is twofold. In the first place, 'delusive' and 'veridical' are *polar* epistemological terms; so that in order to judge a particular perceptual situation to be 'delusive', we must also be able to recognise 'veridical' perceptions—else the very distinction dissolves, and Dr. Broad's argument with it. And in the second place, while it may be, at least in some cases, that delusive perceptual situations are not distinguishable *on their face* from veridical perceptions, they can be distinguished by antecedent and subsequent perceptual experience. Dr. Broad's insistence upon an *internal* basis for distinction, I argue, is arbitrary and question-begging.

Chapter IV, 'The "Logical Question" and the Alternative Theories', is an evaluation of Dr. Broad's argument that in view of illusions and the different appearances which a physical object presents from different perspectives and under different conditions, what is required, logically, if we try to preserve the common-sense view that the objective constituents of perceptual situations are literally parts of the surfaces of external physical objects, is 'a reconsideration of the formal characteristics of the relation of such attributes as size, shape and colour to objective constituents and to physical objects'. He presents two alternative 'theories', 'neither of which accords very well with common sense'. These are, first: the *Theory of Multiple Inherence*, which meets the problem by postulating that sensible characteristics, such as shape, size, and colour, are not 'intrinsic' properties of physical objects, but rather characteristics the specification of which involves an 'essential reference' to a 'region of projection'; and second: the *Multiple Relation Theory of Appearing*, which meets the problem by holding that 'objective constituents can have qualities which are different from and inconsistent with those which they seem on careful inspection to have'. My argument in this chapter is directed toward showing that the 'logical' problem which Dr. Broad generates about illusions and the different appearances of a physical object is not a real problem at all. Contrary to his contention, I insist that the well-known principles of geometric perspective, the behaviour of light, and the nature of the human eye are not only not

31

irrelevant considerations, but do in fact adequately account for the observed facts. The two 'theories', I maintain moreover, are not *factually* alternative with respect to each other or to the common-sense view, but are merely alternative *notational systems* for rendering the observed facts. But ordinary common-sense usage naturally and implicitly embraces such facts as the relevance of the observer and his position, etc., to the apparent characteristics of physical objects. The attempt to reword common expressions to take explicit cognizance of these facts only leads to confusion. Such language as Dr. Broad wants to employ in doing this ordinarily expresses states of affairs which are quite different from the familiar veridical perceptual situations of everyday life, and its use in such cases is either misleading or unintelligible.

In *Chapter V* I discuss Dr. Broad's parallel 'Causal Question'. Such considerations as mirror-images, non-homogeneous media, the finite velocity of light, colour-blindness, morbid bodily states like jaundice, and the effects of drugs like santonin, lead him to conclude that the 'independently necessary and sufficient' material conditions for a certain shade of colour to 'pervade' (or a certain sensible shape and size to 'inform') a certain 'external region' from a certain 'region of projection' are all contained in or close to the 'region of projection'. Here again my argument is concerned with showing that such considerations as Dr. Broad adduces do not pose any problem for our common-sense beliefs and expressions about physical objects and perception. Quite the contrary, they are, in the main, well-known anomalies, and neither their existence nor their explanation is incompatible with the so-called common-sense view. The finite velocity of light, while perhaps not a commonly-known or considered fact, plays no appreciable rôle in the vast majority of ordinary perceptual situations; and in any event it does not enter into the ordinary meaning of our judgment that the objects we see are present before our eyes at the time we see them. Analysis of what he means by the key phrases (in quotation marks above) reveals that for the most part Dr. Broad's conclusion concerning the causal conditions of perception seems contrary to common sense only because of his peculiar choice of language. Some of his generalizations from abnormal perceptual situations, however, reflect his 'Principle of Exceptional Cases' (discussed earlier in this *Introduction*), and are, as I try to show, unwarranted.

INTRODUCTION

Chapter VI, which concludes the essay, is concerned with Dr. Broad's '*Sensum Theory*', the third and favoured solution which he proposes to meet the 'logical problem'. This 'theory' is supposed to meet the 'problem' by abandoning altogether the common-sense view that the objective constituents of veridical perceptual experiences are literally spatio-temporal parts of 'external' physical objects, holding rather that they are unique objects, 'neither mental nor physical', but 'particular existents of a peculiar kind'—*sensa*. Dr. Broad's arguments designed to show that it is 'highly plausible' to take this view are essentially the same as those considered in Chapter IV in connection with the initial statement of the 'logical problem', and are as easily dispatched. As with the other two 'alternative theories', moreover, analysis shows that the Sensum Theory is a purely verbal 'solution' to the pseudo-problem about the multiple appearances which physical objects present; but in addition a certain *reductio ad absurdum* of this theory is shown, stemming from the fact, acknowledged by Dr. Broad, that we do not ordinarily notice any discrepancy between our 'objective constituents' and the physical objects we claim to perceive 'directly'. Finally, I argue that the problem he finds in the familiar fact that objects look different from different perspectives, his insistence that the scientific explanation does not satisfactorily reconcile these different 'appearances' with the common-sense notion of a single, unchanging, 'directly perceived' physical object, and lastly, his preference among the three 'alternative theories' he proposes, all indicate that Dr. Broad implicitly regards the 'objective constituents' of our perceptual experience from the outset as though they were intervening 'entities', like photographic images, or 'sensa'. And in fact, I conclude, Dr. Broad's very sense-datum approach, with its artificial separation between 'directly perceived objective constituents' and 'external physical objects', constitutes nothing less than a tacit assumption of the major premise of the Sensum Theory, and thus foredooms the inquiry to his sceptical conclusions and paradoxical 'theories'.

CHAPTER I

THE 'FACTS' OF PERCEPTION

I

EVERYONE, whatever his philosophical views may be, says Dr. Broad,[1] would admit that such phrases as 'I see a bell', 'I feel a bell', 'I hear a bell' indicate states of affairs which actually exist from time to time. Some people would raise doubts about the existence of physical objects, such as chairs, tables, bells, etc. Some would raise doubts about the existence of selves or minds which perceive such objects. But no one doubts that such phrases as those above express propositions which are sometimes true. People do not begin to quarrel until they try to *analyse* such situations, and to ask what must be meant by 'I', by the 'bell', and by 'hearing', if it is to be true that 'I hear a bell'. And when they do this, he says, they are liable to find that the only senses of 'I', 'bell', and 'hear' which will make the statement true are very different from those which we are wont to attach to these words.

If this should happen, it still remains true, of course, that the phrases 'I hear a bell' and 'I see a chair' stand for real states of affairs which differ in certain specific ways from each other; but these states of affairs may be extremely different in their structure and their components from what the form of words which is used to indicate them would naturally suggest to us.[2]

Before this can be discussed and determined, however, before attempting, that is, any particular *analysis* of them, with which it is

---

1 *The Mind and Its Place in Nature*, pp. 140 ff. (Cf. *Scientific Thought*, p. 236.)
2 *Idem*, p. 140.

certain many people will violently disagree, says Dr. Broad, it is important, here as always, to state the *facts* in a form to which everyone will agree. In endeavouring to accomplish this, Dr. Broad makes certain distinctions to which he affixes special names. Before giving an account of some of these, however, I want to stress again the observations which I set forth in the *Introduction* regarding the preceding suggestion.

I do not think that anyone can reasonably quarrel with Dr. Broad when he says that such phrases as 'I see a bell', 'I feel a bell', 'I hear a bell', and so on indicate states of affairs which actually exist from time to time. That such phrases have a use in everyday life is a matter of common observation. Now the very fact of their having a use in everyday life tells us that they sometimes express true propositions. For they originated in the context of social communication, and their correct usage is determined within that context. They mean nothing more nor less than the kind of experienceable situations to which they were devised to refer. Not *all* propositions of this sort could be always false, for then the sentences which express them would neither have a current usage, nor would they have arisen in our language.

What is more, if the very denial that these phrases express true propositions is ever to have sense, it cannot be the case that they *always* express false propositions. To say that a proposition of this kind is false must mean that the situation indicated is not in fact exemplified. But to determine this, we must first know at least the *kind* of situation which would make such a proposition true, and then see that the actual situation does not conform. Now with propositions of so fundamental a type as these, there is no other way to gain acquaintance with the kind of situation which would make them true than to experience situations of just that kind. Thus it cannot be meaningful to say that the propositions which such phrases express are always false.

It is apparent, however, that though I am in agreement thus far with Dr. Broad that such statements as 'I see a bell' are sometimes true, it is not because he accepts the kind of argument I have advanced. For by the same argument I am forced to disagree with his further statement that when people try to *analyse* such situations as are expressed by these statements, and to ask what is meant by 'I', by 'bell', and by 'hear', if it is to be true that I hear a bell, 'they are liable to find that the only sense of "I", "bell", and "hear" which will make the statement true are very different from those which we are wont to attach to these words'. I find it impossible to accept such a statement even prior to an examination of the arguments which he advances in support of it. Nothing is more clear and certain than that these statements *in their ordinary usage* are often both true and known to be so.

Just as is the case with the statements in which they occur, these words originated in the social context of communication, and their correct usage or meaning is determined within that context. Just as it is inconceivable that a proposition of the type 'I hear a bell' should always be false, so it is inconceivable that such words as 'I', 'bell', and 'hear' which express the proposition should mean something other than we have always understood them to mean. They mean what they were coined to mean; and if the proposition which they express is true, then these words, by the same token, refer to what is the case. Thus, any arguments which claim to deny this must *ipso facto* be false or sophistical. What those arguments are, and at what point they go astray, I shall try to show in subsequent chapters. But the preceding comments may be taken, in general, as an indication of the line which the subsequent discussion and criticism will follow.

2

Such situations as are naturally indicated by phrases like 'I am seeing a chair' or 'I am hearing a bell' Dr. Broad refers to as 'Perceptual Situations'. That there are such situations everyone agrees. 'Can we all agree to go any further together before parting company?' Dr. Broad thinks we obviously can. He asks us to consider the following three statements:

1. I am hearing a bell.
2. I am seeing pink rats. (Delusive.)
3. I feel cross.

When we consider statements of the third kind, says Dr. Broad, we realize that they differ radically from the first or perceptual kind. When we feel cross, he observes, we are not feeling some-*thing* but are feeling some*how*. When we hear a bell, we no doubt, he says, are feeling some*how*; but the important thing about the perceptual situation is that we 'claim to be in cognitive contact with some*thing* other than ourselves and our states'. This claim is just as obvious in those perceptual situations which are commonly believed to be delusive, he observes, as in those which are commonly believed to be veridical. The situation 'I feel cross', however, differs from the other two which are alike in this respect. This difference Dr. Broad expresses by saying that the first two do, and the third does not, have an 'epistemological object'. The bell situation and the pink-rat situation both have epistemological objects; the situation indicated by 'I feel cross' has no epistemological object.

My motive in adding the qualifying word 'epistemological' is that otherwise some bright spirit will at once complain that the pink-rat situation has no object. What he really means is of course that there is no *ontological* object, corresponding to the *epistemological* object which the situation certainly has; i.e., that the situation involves a certain claim which the physical world refuses to meet.[1]

At this point, I want to comment on the distinction which Dr. Broad has made between 'epistemological object' and 'ontological object' with respect to perceptual situations. Now the difference between perceptual and non-perceptual situations, which is expressed in terms of having or not having an epistemological object, is that in the one case—the perceptual situation—there is the claim to 'cognitive contact with some*thing* other than ourselves and our states'; whereas in the non-perceptual situation—'I feel cross', etc.—there is not this claim. The difference, then, which Dr. Broad is taking note of is one of claims, and not, so far, one involving similarity or difference in the number of entities which are actually to be distinguished in the analysis of the three situations. That is to say, what situations of the kind 'I am seeing a rat' (or "I am hearing a bell", where these are veridical), and situations of the kind 'I am seeing pink rats' (delusive) have in common, is only that they make similar claims concerning cognitive contact with something other than ourselves and our states, and not any common entity perceived in both cases.

But this difference and similarity in *claims* is misleadingly expressed by Dr. Broad as though the non-perceptual situation

1 *Idem*, pp. 141 f.

differed from the other two, the veridical and delusive perceptual situations, in that the latter two had some*thing* in common beside the claim, namely an 'epistemological *object*'. This way of stating the 'facts' paves the way for the analysis of delusive 'perceptual' situations in terms of 'cognitive contact' with a kind of 'particular'. When we come to Dr. Broad's analysis of the 'facts' we find that the particular has become a kind of *existent*, neither mental nor physical. And eventually Dr. Broad's analysis of even veridical perception involves such an entity intervening, whether logically or substantially, between the perceiver and the physical object which he perceives. All this derives from, or at least is given a surface plausibility by, the leap which Dr. Broad makes from the statement that delusive as well as veridical perceptions make or contain the claim to cognitive contact, to the statement that they both 'have epistemological objects'.

On Dr. Broad's own definition of how he proposes to use the term 'epistemological object', it seems to me, he should have no quarrel with the 'bright spirit' who complains that the pink-rat situation really has no object. For the latter in making his complaint is certainly not unaware of, and does not mean to deny, the 'claim' which delusive perceptions, on their face, seem to make. Nor is he unaware of the difference between experiences like 'I feel cross' and perceptual situations of the veridical and delusive types. What he 'really means' by his complaint is just what he says: that there is no object in the pink-rat situation. Dr. Broad evades this point when he speaks of an 'epistemological object'. The very importance which he places on this way of putting the matter belies his statement that he is expressing only a similarity in claims when he says that both veridical and delusive perceptual situations 'have epistemological objects'.

Dr. Broad has defined 'epistemological object' in terms of the claim to external cognitive contact which characterizes perceptual situations, both hallucinatory and veridical. Now consider the case when one has an hallucinatory or hallucinatory-like experience, and knows at the time that it is not veridical. On Dr. Broad's explanation of the term, it is not at all clear that such a situation involves an 'epistemological object'. For when the individual knows that his experience is not veridical, then it is not true that he is making any claim to external cognitive contact. Dr. Broad vacillates between saying that it is *we* who make this claim which characterizes all perceptual situations,[1] and that it is the *situation* which 'involves' the claim, or 'has' an epistemological object.[2] But situations do not make such claims; it is of course we who make them. In what sense, then, can an hallucinatory perceptual situation which is recognized as such by the perceiver be said to involve the claim to external cognitive contact? What Dr. Broad must mean, it seems to me, is merely that the hallucinatory experience bears a subjective resemblance to the veridical perceptual experience which would correspond in its descriptive qualitative aspects if one were actually perceiving an external physical object or phenomenon. Perceptual situations are situations involving sensory experience in any of the modalities through which we do have external cognitive contact with physical objects or phenomena: sight, sound, touch, taste, and smell. A situation may be classified as perceptual so long as it involves experiences in these modalities, whether the experience is veridical or hallucinatory. Dr. Broad, then, might better say that a perceptual situation has an epistemological object if it involves a sensory experience which is qualitatively like the experience which the subject would have if he were actually perceiving a corresponding physical object or phenomenon.

In what sense of the term 'object' may hallucinatory perceptual situations be said to have objects? Compare the two situations 'I am seeing pink rats' (delusive) and 'I am seeing a rat' (veridical). In the veridical perception the rat that is seen is a physical object. But when one is having the delusion of 'seeing pink rats', obviously there are no such rats being perceived. Nevertheless, he is having a visual experience which is very much like that he has when he actually sees a rat. And it is natural, for grammatical reasons, to refer to the descriptive content of this kind of experience *as though* it were actually an object that was being revealed. Thus, we may only in an analogous and purely grammatical sense speak of the 'objects' of our hallucinatory experiences.

But now, in view of what has just been said, we may ask if there

---

[1] Cf. *idem*, p. 141: '. . . The important point about the perceptual situation is that we claim to be in cognitive contact with some*thing* other than ourselves and our states.'

[2] Cf. *idem*, p. 142: 'What he really means is of course that there is no *ontological* object, corresponding to the *epistemological* object which the situation certainly has: i.e., that the situation involves a certain claim which the physical world refuses to meet.'

is any justification for the use of the term 'epistemological object' in the case of veridical perceptions. When it is true that 'I am seeing a rat', there is a physical object which is *the* object which I am seeing. It is literally an object, and not an object in a sense only analogous to some other, as in the previous case. This is the primary sense of the word 'object' to which its use in cases of delusive perception is only analogous. The two cases, then, have no common object. The veridical situation involves an object, but the delusive situation involves only an experience which is subjectively very much like—though objectively very much unlike—that which one has of an object. The fact that both experiences may involve the same subjective claim—or at least the absence of doubt—as to veridicality, does not alter the objective difference between the two situations. There is good reason, then, to consider 'epistemological object' (if this be more than the claim to veridicality) and 'ontological object' as mutually exclusive terms. For when what one is describing is a physical object (in veridical perception), there is no ground for his speaking also of an 'epistemological *object*', by which, as we have seen, Dr. Broad seems to mean not simply the claim to veridicality, but the visual sensation itself, hypostatized into a kind of entity. Thus far, at least, in what purports to be a statement of the facts with which everyone can agree, Dr. Broad has not shown that there is any basis, in the veridical perception of an object, for distinguishing the 'experiential content' from the object itself.

3

In connection with the objections advanced in the preceding section, Dr. Broad seems to have something to say in his own defence:

I had better take this opportunity to anticipate another purely verbal objection which someone is sure to make. Someone is certain to say: 'We don't really *see* pink rats, for there are none; we only think we see them.' To this I answer by admitting that words like 'seeing', 'hearing', etc., do, most unfortunately, introduce the 'fallacy of many questions' like the barrister's query: 'When did you leave off beating your wife?' The phrase 'I see so-and-so' *is* taken in ordinary life to mean: 'There is a perceptual situation of the visual kind of which I am subject. This has such and such an epistemological object. And there is a physical object corresponding to this epistemological object.' If a second person has reason to believe that the third of these propositions is false, he will be inclined to say: 'You are not really seeing so-and-so; you only think that you are seeing it'. Now words like 'seeing' and 'hearing' are hopeless for our present purpose if they are to be interpreted in this way. I therefore wish it to be clearly understood that I shall depart so far from common usage as to say that a man *sees* a pink rat, provided he is subject of a perceptual situation which has a pink rat as an epistemological object and is of the visual kind, regardless of whether there is a physical pink rat corresponding to this epistemological object.[1]

In this section I want to discuss Dr. Broad's explanation of the terminology he employs in dealing with veridical and hallucinatory perceptual experience, and incidentally to explain the terminology which I myself shall henceforth employ.

I have already commented on Dr. Broad's use of the term 'epistemological object'. With respect to the quotation above, I can only repeat that the phrase 'I see so-and-so' is not taken in ordinary life to mean: 'There is a perceptual situation of the visual kind. This has an epistemological object, etc.' I suggest that what the phrase 'I see so-and-so' means might better be put: 'There is a so-and-so and I see it.' If 'epistemological object' means no more than the claim to external cognitive contact, the substitute meaning which I offer ought to be perfectly acceptable to Dr. Broad; for it expresses the claim equally well, and certainly more typically. Why is Dr. Broad not content to explain merely that he proposes to say that a man *sees* a pink rat even when he is only having an hallucination? Why should he insist on the 'epistemological object' way of putting it?

Now what about Dr. Broad's apology for departing so far from common usage as to say that a man *sees* pink rats, even when his experience is hallucinatory and there are no such rats? The fact is that there seems to be no explicit convention in ordinary language concerning the use of such terms as 'perceive', 'see', 'feel', 'hear', and so forth, with respect to the distinction between veridical and non-veridical or hallucinatory experience. Certainly in the greater number of instances in which we ordinarily have occasion to employ these terms, our intention is to assert or refer to a veridical experience. Ordinarily, when we say 'I see a chair' (or etc.), we mean that there is a physical object

[1] *Idem*, p. 142.

of a certain kind before us, and that we are experiencing it visually. Under certain circumstances, the primary intention of an 'I see . . .' (or an 'I saw . . .') proposition may be to call attention to the sense modality in or through which the object is (or was) perceived. But usually, I believe, our interest is primarily in reporting the presence of the object, or our awareness of its presence, and not in emphasizing the particular sense-modality involved. The fact of illusory and hallucinatory sensory experiences, however, provides a complication.

From the subjective point of view, hallucinatory experiences, whether recognized as such or not, do bear a similarity to veridical experiences, just as the buzz which is heard when there is a short circuit in a telephone switchboard is superficially not distinguishable from the buzz which is produced when there is actually a call coming in from the outside. The after-image which one experiences when he closes his eyes after looking intently at a bright light is recognized as a visual or 'seeing' experience. Thus, it is natural to extend the meaning of the term 'see' from visual awareness of an external object to merely the having of a visual experience. To reserve perceptual terms for veridical experiences only would, as Dr. Broad justifiably insists, involve us in awkward circumlocutions. It is natural to report hallucinatory experiences in the same terms we use to describe the objects which we perceive in veridical experiences, even when we are aware that our experiences are hallucinatory. The alcoholic who does not question his experience reports that he 'sees' pink rats; but even when he is free from the hallucination and is capable of judging his experience as having been delusive, it is natural for him to say that he 'saw' pink rats while under the influence of alcohol. While sometimes we circumvent this difficulty by employing a phrase like 'I *thought* I saw . . .,' etc., this is not altogether satisfactory. For it suggests more than is intended, and what is not usually the case, namely, that at the time one had such an experience he consciously and explicitly affirmed to himself that his experience was veridical. What is undoubtedly closer to the truth is that most individuals having such experiences do not at the time consciously question their veridicality at all, but merely take them as veridical without consideration.

Now Dr. Broad proposes to employ terms like 'see' and 'feel' to mean merely 'to have a visual experience' and 'to have a tactual experience'. In this way he is able to allow the fact of such experiences without prejudicing the discussion of whether or not there exist corresponding 'ontological objects'. Thus, he can speak of '*seeing* pink rats'. I want to make clear that my quarrel here is not with this decision concerning the use of terms, as such, which has the justification of convenience. Rather I am questioning the justification for the classification of the pink-rat type of experience with veridical visual experience on the assumption that, being both 'perceptual', they will yield similar analyses into an act of perceiving and an 'epistemological object', with the addition of 'ontological object' in the case of veridical perception. It is this assumption which I contend goes beyond the 'facts with which everyone will agree'. As I shall show in later chapters, this type of false bifurication between 'epistemological objects' and 'ontological object' in the case of veridical perception is a practice which lends a specious plausibility to the Sensum Theory of perception.

In introducing the notion of 'epistemological object', Dr. Broad called attention to the difference between such statements as 'I am hearing a bell' (or 'I am seeing a rat'—i.e., veridical experiences) and 'I am seeing pink rats' (delusive), on the one hand, and statements of the kind 'I feel cross'. The difference, he said, was that statements of the first kind claim cognitive contact, with some*thing* other than ourselves and our states, while those of the latter kind do not make this claim. It is on the basis of the similarity of claims, then, that Dr. Broad chooses to group veridical and delusive visual experiences as 'perceptual'. The justification for the use of the term 'see' in both the veridical and delusive cases is apparently that they are both experiences of the visual kind. I do not mean to deny the possibility of this type of classification. But I do want to call attention to the fact that on the basis of the realization of, or the failure in realizing, the claim to cognitive contact with some*thing* other than ourselves and our states, an equally defensible classification would be to group hallucinatory visual experiences with the non-perceptual, in which group in this respect they clearly fall. The kind of situation which Dr. Broad calls non-perceptual differs from both veridical and delusive perceptual situations in that it makes no *claim* to external cognitive contact. But delusive visual experiences are like the non-perceptual in that neither do *in fact* reveal any *thing* other than ourselves and our states. Regardless of which arrangement is made, the important thing is to see clearly in just what respects delusive visual experiences are like the veridical perceptual, and in what respects like the non-perceptual, and to bear these likenesses and differences in mind for future reference.

I want to take this opportunity to explain my own use of perceptual terminology. As a matter of fact, there seems to be little general consistency in the use of the term 'perception' itself even among philosophers. In more or less accord with popular usage, Runes' *Dictionary of Philosophy*[1] defines perception, in the sense with which we are concerned, as 'the apprehension of ordinary sense-objects, such as trees, houses, chairs, etc., on the occasion of sensory stimulation'. But the same work defines hallucination as 'a non-veridical or delusive perception of a sense object occurring when no object is in fact present to the organs of sense'. It is clear that if consistency were observed, an hallucination, not being 'the apprehension of an ordinary sense-object . . . on the occasion of sensory stimulation', could not properly be said to be a perception at all.

Technical usage does seem, however, to have established different meanings for the terms 'hallucination' and 'illusion'. The distinction reflected by these terms seems to be this: a perceptual experience is said to be an *illusion* if it involves a misinterpretation of the data of sense, where such data are actually present to the external sense organs. An illusion is the result of unusual conditions of perception, physical, physiological, and/or psychological. Examples of illusions are the taking of a configuration of shrubs in the garden for the figure of a man, or the misjudgment of the relative sizes of objects in unusual juxtapositions, or the bent appearance of a straight stick when it is immersed half in water and half in air. A sensory experience is said to be an *hallucination* if instead of involving merely misinterpretation of given external stimuli, it arises wholly internally. What it seems to reveal about the immediate physical environment is either not even remotely the case, or, if it happens to be, is *causally* irrelevant to the experience.

Borderline cases immediately come to mind for a decision. For

---

[1] Dagobert D. Runes, ed. (1942); the definitions of 'perception' and 'hallucination' were contributed by Ledger Wood.

44

example, when one presses on his eyeball with his fingers, a visual experience—perhaps a sensation of colour—may result. Such an experience is clearly the result of an external stimulus. However, although for psychiatric purposes it is not sufficiently pathological to warrant being termed an hallucination, for our purposes it is better classified as such. For such an experience does not reveal, in the normal, directly causal fashion, the visual characteristics of the stimulating object. The visual experience resulting from pressure on the eyeball can hardly be termed a visual experience of the finger which is pressing. On the other hand, in certain pathological mental states, normal sensory stimulation by an external object may give rise to a visual experience so totally irrelevant to the actual descriptive qualities of the stimulating object as to demand classification as hallucinatory.

The common after-image experience which occurs when one closes his eyes after looking intently at a bright light is another borderline case. Here the experience results from the over-stimulation of a sense organ, with a persistence of effect after the external stimulus is removed. In view of the spatial and temporal proximity, and the direct causal relationship between the external stimulus and the after-image experience, there seems to be justification for speaking of it as 'illusory'. On the other hand, its occurrence in the immediate absence of any relevant external stimulus seems to warrant its classification as hallucinatory.

In view of the absence of consistent usage, and the foregoing considerations, I propose to adopt the following terminology. I do not mean to suggest that it is an ideal usage which I am proposing, but offer it only as an expedient toward clarity of communication in making the distinctions I want to make. In this paper I shall follow Dr. Broad's example in employing such terms as 'perception', 'perceptual', 'sensory', 'see', 'hear', 'visual', 'tactual', etc., in such a way as to refer only to the subjective aspect of experience, without prejudice to the question of whether or not the particular experience is veridical. Thus, 'I see a chair' and 'I see pink rats' will both be termed visual and perceptual. Where I require to distinguish between the two possible cases, I shall employ the terms 'normal' or 'veridical' and 'hallucinatory' or 'non-veridical'. By a 'normal' or 'veridical' visual perception, for instance, I am going to mean the familiar kind of experience which the reader would normally understand by such propositions as

45

'I see a chair', 'I see the moon', etc. That is, I shall mean to refer, in the sense in which these words are ordinarily understood, to those situations in which an individual in the normal sensory fashion perceives a chair, or the moon, etc., through his eyes, where such physical objects are actually present and visible. By a non-veridical perception I shall mean an experience of the hallucinatory type, adhering to the distinction between hallucination and illusion set forth above. Moreover, I propose to classify after-image experiences and such experiences as the visual experiences resulting from pressing on the eyeball with the finger, as hallucinatory. Finally, for the purposes of this essay, I shall maintain the distinction between the terms 'illusion' and 'hallucination' as given above, and I shall limit the meaning of 'non-veridical' to the latter type of experience. I do this because of my contention that the analysis of situations of the former type does involve external, physical objects and objective conditions of perception, as does the analysis of normal veridical perceptual situations.

4

Omitting, as not immediately relevant to the discussion in succeeding chapters, the intervening distinctions which Dr. Broad makes between situations which are held to be perceptual and those which are not, I want to turn to the last of the points which he supposes everyone would admit to be common and peculiar to the former. This, he says, is the fact that sensation plays a unique and indispensable part in them. He writes:

I do not think it is possible to define 'sensations'. But it is possible to give illustrations which everyone will recognize. Such statements as 'I am aware of a red flash', 'I am aware of a squeaky noise', and so on, are certainly sometimes true; and they express a kind of situation which is perfectly familiar to everyone. Whenever such a statement is true, there exists a sensation. And it would be admitted that there cannot be perceptual situations without sensations. I think that it would also be admitted sensations play a part in perceptual situations which they do not play in any other kind of situation. I will express this fact by saying that perceptual situations are 'sensuous'.[1]

I want to try to get clear as to just what it is that Dr. Broad

---

[1] *The Mind and Its Place in Nature*, p. 145.

means by 'sensation'. Even if he is right in holding that the term cannot be *defined*, it is important to determine at least the kind of thing he means by it, so that we may decide whether or not what he says about it is true. Different philosophers and psychologists have used the term in different ways, and certainly not all of these usages would evoke the kind of agreement which Dr. Broad claims for his assertions. I assume that Dr. Broad means to say more than merely that everyone would employ the *word* 'sensation' in connection with perceptual situations, whatever they might mean by it. What, then, does Dr. Broad intend by this term?

Now I do not find it at all clear from Dr. Broad's remarks here just which aspects of the situations expressed by statements such as 'I am aware of a red flash', 'I am aware of a squeaky noise', his use of the term 'sensation' refers to. It is not clear just why Dr. Broad supposes that whenever it is true that 'I am aware of a red flash', a sensation exists. Is this intended to be merely a definition by partial denotation, and is 'being aware of a red flash' itself the sort of thing Dr. Broad would call a sensation? Or would he consider this to be a perceptual situation in which a sensation 'plays a part'? In that case, which aspect of the situation is the sensation? If 'being aware of a red flash' is a perceptual situation, is it then an empirical proposition that whenever such a situation exists, there exists *also* a sensation? If what Dr. Broad means by a 'sensation' is simply a specific physiological excitation of the sensory apparatus or nervous system, then he is quite right in saying that everyone would agree that sensation plays a unique and indispensable part in perceptual situations. For regardless of whether a perceptual situation is veridical or hallucinatory, it is certain that some modification of the nervous system is involved; and it is likely that the sort of modification that is involved in perceptual situations is different from the sort which is involved in other types of mental experience.

There is reason to suppose, however, that this is not what Dr. Broad has in mind when he employs the term 'sensation'. In explaining what he means by a *perceptual situation* Dr. Broad, as we have seen, gives such examples as 'I see a *chair*' and 'I hear a *bell*'; while in explaining what he means by *sensation*, he refers only to 'being aware of a red flash' and 'being aware of a squeaky noise'. If all that he meant by a sensation was physiological stimulation, he could have referred again to his original examples. For the existence of the physiological process is as much a fact in the former examples as it is in the latter. The fact that he did choose different types of examples does seem to indicate that he means to denote a distinction between perception and sensation; and it also suggests that the distinction does not have to do with physiology.

Now in contemporary psychology and epistemology, 'perception' is usually defined as the apprehension of ordinary sense objects, such as trees, houses, chairs, etc., in distinction to 'sensation', which refers to the apprehension of isolated sense qualities: coloured patches, noises, smells, etc.[1] If this is the distinction which Dr. Broad has in mind, then 'being aware of a red flash' and 'being aware of a squeaky noise' would be examples of sensations. Unfortunately, in order to ascertain whether or not we are correct in supposing this to be the distinction that Dr. Broad means to make, I must anticipate somewhat his subsequent analysis of the facts, with which, as he says himself, philosophers are apt to quarrel. (Happily, however, this will also afford an opportunity to discuss briefly certain relevant topics which are not dealt with in subsequent chapters.)

Dr. Broad analyses sensation as an 'act of sensing' directed upon a kind of 'particular concrete existent', which he calls a 'sensum'. Thus, he writes:

When a man talks of a 'sensation of red', he is sometimes referring to a red patch which he senses, sometimes to his act of sensing the patch, and sometimes to the whole complex state of affairs, which, on the sensum theory, is analysable into (act of sensing)—directed on to —(red patch). In the second meaning, 'sensation' is obviously mental; in the third it is undoubtedly a complex whole which involves a mental factor. In the first meaning, it is by no means obvious or even plausible to say that a sensation is mental. I shall always use 'sensation' in the third meaning.[2]

And elsewhere he says:

Under certain conditions I have states of mind called sensations. These sensations have objects, which are always concrete particular existents, like coloured or hot patches, noises, smells, etc. Such objects

[1] Cf. Runes, *Dictionary of Philosophy*, p. 228; the contribution 'Perception' is by Ledger Wood.
[2] *Scientific Thought*, p. 249.

are called sensa. Sensa have properties, such as shape, size, hardness, colour, loudness, coldness, and so on. The existence of such sensa, and their presence to our minds in sensation, lead us to judge that a physical object exists and is present to our senses.[1]

Now from these two passages, we might suppose that Dr. Broad clearly means that the experience of being aware of a simple isolated quality like colour, sound, etc., is itself a sensation. And thus we might suppose that there is no question but that 'being aware of a red flash' and 'being aware of a squeaky noise', being both experiences of this sort, are examples of sensations. But subsequently Dr. Broad writes as though he were in agreement with those psychologists and epistemologists who hold that we never experience sensations as such, but only perceptions, and that, hence, 'being aware of a red flash' would not be a sensation, but rather a perception.

A distinguishable feature in perceptual situations, he writes,[2] is that certain specific bodily feelings, certain emotions, and certain feelings of expectation (causally dependent on the traces left by past experience) are related in a unique way to the apprehended sensum. When a sensum of a specific kind is intuitively apprehended, certain traces are excited which arouse certain emotions and induce bodily adjustments which are accompanied by bodily feelings. In addition, even if it does not call up specific images, the apprehension of a sensum may at least evoke a more or less vague feeling of 'familiarity'. These 'mnemic consequences' of the apprehension of the sensum, moreover, do not merely coexist with it, but immediately enter into a specific kind of relation to it which, Dr. Broad tells us, he does not know how to analyse further. These 'mnemic consequences' in this specific relation to

---

[1] *Idem*, p. 243. It must be remembered that Dr. Broad has said that he will use the terms and phrases of language about perception in such a way as not to assume cognitive contact with external reality. Thus, in this quotation, and in the one just preceding, Dr. Broad means to say that such concrete, particular, non-mental existents which he calls 'sensa' would exist in *any* perceptual situation, whether it was veridical or purely hallucinatory. (It may be noted that in this quotation Dr. Broad refers to sensations as 'states of mind', while in the passage quoted just above he explicitly states that it is only the 'act of sensing' which is mental, and that he will always use 'sensation' to refer to the whole complex process which is not itself mental, but only involves a mental factor. This inconsistency may perhaps be due to the fact that the second quotation occurs in the text itself *earlier* than the first quotation—that is, before Dr. Broad announces his resolution to employ the term in this strict sense.)

[2] *The Mind and Its Place in Nature*, p. 215.

this intuitively apprehended sensum constitute what he calls the 'quasi-belief' about the sensum which, he says, gives the situation its specific 'External Reference'.[1]

These considerations lead Dr. Broad to discuss precisely the issue with which we are concerned. But his answer only involves us in further uncertainty as to what, exactly, a sensation, as such, is. He writes:

Can there be pure sensation without perception? Let us see exactly what this means on our theory. A pure sensation would be a situation in which a certain sensum, e.g., a noise or a coloured patch, was intuitively apprehended, but in which there was no external reference. Now, on our theory, we should expect perception to melt into pure sensation by insensible degrees; we should expect the latter to be an ideal limit rather than an observable fact; and we should expect it to be unstable and transitory, if it happens at all. If the mass of feeling be highly differentiated and certain specific parts of it be specifically related to a certain sensum, we shall have a clear case of perceptual situation with a definite external reference. If, on the other hand, the mass of feeling be little differentiated, and the apprehension of the sensum fails to excite traces which cause specific modifications in the mass, we shall have a situation which approximates to pure sensation, since its external reference will be very vague. And the same result would happen, even if the mass of feeling were differentiated in the way suggested, provided that for some reason the differentiated parts fail to enter into the proper relation to the apprehended sensum. It seems to me that when we are looking at something with interest our awareness of the sensa towards the edge of the visual field approximates to pure sensation for the first reason. And, perhaps, when we are looking for something and discover afterwards that it was staring us in the face all the time, our awareness of the sensa connected with it approximates to pure sensation from the second cause.[2]

It is obvious that this passage returns us to a state of indecision

---

[1] By the 'external reference' of the perceptual situation, Dr. Broad means a disposition to respond to the given sensed sensum as though it were literally part of a certain larger and persistent external physical object or event. It seems to be the same thing as what he originally referred to in terms of the phrase 'epistemological object', the 'claim to be in cognitive contact with some*thing* other than ourselves and our states'. He speaks of a 'quasi-belief' about this to indicate that he does not mean an explicit belief or judgment involving inference from sensum to external object, but rather an automatic attitude or expectation, which occurs whether the situation is veridical or hallucinatory, and even when the subject is intellectually aware that it is hallucinatory.

[2] *The Mind and Its Place in Nature*, p. 216.

as to whether Dr. Broad means to offer 'being aware of a red flash' and 'being aware of a squeaky noise' as examples of sensations which 'play a part in' perceptual situations, or as examples of perceptual situations in which sensations play a part. Though previously he spoke of having a visual experience of red as being a sensation, it would seem from this discussion that 'being aware of a red flash' or 'being aware of a squeaky noise' are really perceptions. For neither of these cases approximate the conditions which Dr. Broad sets forth in this passage for being a pure sensation. What is experienced in the situation indicated by the phrase 'being aware of a red flash', for instance, is experienced *as* red, *as* a flash, *as* bright or dim. Moreover, it is recognized as being visual; and even if it be the kind of experience which occurs when we bump our heads in the dark, and it is known to be purely hallucinatory, it does *look* as though there were something 'out there', as Dr. Broad himself argued above. All these factors clearly make the situation perceptual, on Dr. Broad's own criteria. If even so simple an experience as 'being aware of a red flash' is a perception, we may wonder just what, exactly, the sensation is that 'plays a part in' this perceptual situation.

But Dr. Broad does not even consistently maintain this second position. For he subsequently returns to his former and apparently contradictory stand that we are capable of experiencing sensations as such. He urges that we must, 'in the most ordinary statement' about a physical object which we perceive, distinguish between the perception itself and the sensation on which it is based. And he seems quite clearly to mean not that we can do this only theoretically, but that we can actually isolate and attend to the sensation as such, apart from the perception. A perception of a chair, he says, is based on sensations of certain interrelated sensa which are an appearance of it.[1] These sensations, he holds, would consist of sensing, let us say, a brown patch of such and such a shape, with such and such variations in shade and colour, etc. Though ordinarily, he says, we pass automatically from the sensum and its properties to judgments about physical objects and their properties, in which alone we are interested, we can, when the sensum is queer—as when we see double—or even in normal cases, detect the properties of sensa, and contrast them with those which they are leading us to ascribe to the physical object, provided

1 *Idem*, p. 420.

that we make a special effort of attention. In this vein, he goes on to say:

. . . Sensa have never been objects of special interest, and therefore have never been given a name in common speech. A result of this is that all words like 'seeing', 'hearing', etc., are ambiguous. They stand sometimes for acts of sensing, whose objects are of course sensa, and sometimes for acts of perceiving, whose objects are supposed to be bits of matter and their sensible qualities. This is especially clear about hearing. We talk of 'hearing a noise' and of 'hearing a bell'. In the first case we mean that we are sensing an auditory sensum, with certain attributes of pitch, loudness, quality, etc. In the second case we mean that, in consequence of sensing such a sensum, we judge that a certain physical object exists and is present to our senses. Here the word 'hearing' stands for an act of perceiving. Exactly the same remarks apply to sight. In one case we see a penny; in a somewhat stricter sense we see only one side of the penny; in another sense we see only a brown elliptical sensum. The first two uses refer to acts of perceiving, the last to an act of sensing. It is best on the whole to confine words like 'seeing' and 'hearing' to acts of perceiving. This is, of course, their ordinary use. I shall therefore talk of seeing a penny, but not of seeing a brown elliptical sensum. I shall speak of the latter kind of cognition as 'visually sensing', or merely as 'sensing', when no misunderstanding is to be feared by dropping the adjective. This distinction will be found important when we come to deal with illusory perceptions.[1]

When we recall what Dr. Broad said, in the passage previously quoted, about the automatic, involuntary 'mnemic consequences' of the apprehension of a sensum, which do not merely coexist with it, but immediately enter into a specific kind of relation to it, what Dr. Broad is suggesting here seems to be virtually impossible of achievement. The transformation of the hypothetical sensation into the perception occurs, as he said, in an automatic and involuntary fashion on a level below our intellectual conscious control. And I, for one, find it impossible to place myself in such a primitive state of mind that I can have a visual experience of a patch of colour, for example, without at the same time being aware of at least some of the elements which Dr. Broad has said constitute a perception rather than a sensation. I find this so when I am perceiving a simple sense quality, as when I see a red flash; and especially when I am perceiving a physical object.

[1] *Scientific Thought*, p. 247.

When I perceive a chair, there is nothing which I can distinguish, in the manner which Dr. Broad describes, from the chair, or at least the visible part of the chair, itself. Dr. Broad claims that he can distinguish the visual sensum: brown patch of such and such a shape, etc., which 'plays a part in' the perceptual situation 'seeing a chair', and which leads him to judge that a chair exists and is present to his senses. Now, to be sure, when I see a chair of that colour and shape, it is true that I am seeing a brown patch of colour of such and such a shape, etc. But I cannot agree that the sense in which I see this is a different sense from that in which I see the chair (or at least the immediately visible part of the chair). It is perfectly clear to me that what I am doing when I talk about seeing a brown patch of such and such a shape is describing the appearance of the chair which I see, and not the appearance of something else. At the same time, I realize that it would be a highly inadequate description of what I see, no matter to what degree of detail I carried this type of description. For it would always sound as though what I was seeing was a kind of coloured vapour, or the like, having the general shape of a chair.

In supposing that he can distinguish a brown patch of colour of such and such a shape—a sensum—from the chair itself, in his visual field, Dr. Broad, I suspect, is merely *considering* the chair which he sees *as though* it were only a 'patch of colour', like an after-image. Thus he is able to persuade himself that he is attending to a sensation rather than to a chair. It is as though he were considering his perception of the chair as at the same time veridical and hallucinatory. Thus, when he says he is attending to the sensation, rather than to the perception, he conceives of what he sees as though it were merely an hallucinatory image; and when he says he is attending to the perception, he is considering the same thing which he saw before, only now he has made a mental gesture, as it were, and is considering it as a real chair. In subsequent chapters we shall find that Dr. Broad argues that an hallucination and a veridical visual experience cannot on their face be distinguished from each other. In this way, he finds it plausible to suppose that a kind of hallucinatory image, only 'non-mental', i.e., a *sensum*, is what we really see 'directly' even in cases of veridical perception of physical objects. And from this contention, of course, it is but a short step to the possibility that sensa are 'all that there are', and that physical objects are only 'constructs' or 'categories of experience'.

But here I am anticipating arguments that will be discussed in considerably more detail in later chapters. For the present, we must sum up the results of the investigation thus far, and consider whether or not, in terms of what Dr. Broad means by a 'sensation', we can agree that sensations play a part in perception, and that there cannot be perceptual situations without sensations. We have seen that in all probability Dr. Broad would not want to say that 'being aware of a red flash' or 'being aware of a squeaky noise' are examples of pure sensations; but rather that they are perceptual situations. In fact, it would seem that it is an impossibility to detect a pure sensation as such; and thus, when Dr. Broad claims to be able to do so, in a perceptual situation, what he means, by his own criteria, is that he is able to detect the simple perceptions —that is, the perception of simple, isolated qualities—which lead him, in the total perceptual situation, to judge that he is seeing a physical object.

Can we, however, even on this explanation of what Dr. Broad must mean by a 'sensation', grant that everyone would agree that sensations 'play a part in' perceptual situations, and that there could not be perceptual situations without sensations?

It seems to me, in the first place, that there are instances in which the perception of a simple quality (i.e., *sensation*) does not 'play a part in', but literally *constitutes* the total perceptual situation. An example of such a case would be a visual after-image, or the visual experience of colour we have when we bump our heads in the dark. Either of these experiences may consist of a momentary flash of red. Though we might *know* that we were having an hallucinatory experience, still, as Dr. Broad has himself pointed out, it would look to us as though it were a perception of something 'out there'. This quasi-belief about the external reference of our experience, its *apparent* claim to external cognitive contact, would, on Dr. Broad's criteria, make this a perceptual situation. The same sort of situation might arise even in veridical circumstances if we see a sudden flash of red in a perfectly dark room. Thus, there are at least some situations in which sensations (perceptions of simple qualities) do not play a part in the total perceptual situation, nor lead us to judge that anything *else* is present to our senses, but literally constitute the total perceptual situation.

But now what about our perceptions of complex objects and events? Is it true that everyone would agree that the perception of simple isolated qualities plays an indispensable part in our perception of chairs, tables, and the like? It seems to me to be perfectly obvious that when we see a chair, for example, we do not see merely a sum of simple, isolated qualities; we see a chair. Though in seeing a chair I may notice that it has such and such characteristics, enumeratively, it does not follow that I see them this way. I see a chair from the first; and what I am doing when I enumerate these qualities is describing the chair which I see.

Dr. Broad seems to be perfectly aware of this when he argues against those philosophers who want to 'reduce' what he calls the 'higher terms in the hierarchy of mental factors . . . to the lower terms of this hierarchy'. He writes:

Now it seems to me that this is plainly impossible when we clearly understand what is required. Let us take an example. There is a certain event which has the characteristic of being a perception of a pink rat. Let us make the most favourable assumption possible for the reductive type of theory. Let us suppose that this perception has no existent constituents except events which are feelings and events which are acquaintances with sensa and images. We are to suppose then that this perception consists of such events interrelated in certain characteristic ways, and of nothing else. It seems to me that it would still be impossible to *deduce* from the fact that it has this structure and is composed of these constituents, and from laws which are entirely about *feelings* and *sensations*, that this event will be the *perception* of an epistemological object and that this epistemological object will be a pink rat. Unless we had actually met with events which were perceptions and had epistemological objects I do not see that we could possibly have suspected that a whole composed of feelings and sensations interrelated in certain ways would have the property of being the perception of a certain epistemological object. Thus the characteristic of being a perception is not a reducible characteristic, like the behaviour of a clock, but is at best an emergent characteristic, like the behaviour of silver-chloride.[1]

Now it seems to *me* that what Dr. Broad is conceding with one hand he takes away with the other. He seems to be saying in this quotation that we do have mental experiences which are perceptions as such, and that perceptions as such are not reducible to a

[1] *The Mind and Its Place in Nature*, pp. 638 f.

mere structural interrelation of sensations. Yet he also wants to say that the process of perception is one of going from the sensation of simple qualities to the total perception of objects. Apparently he feels that this seeming contradiction is resolved by conceiving of perception as an *emergent* characteristic of the concatenation of simple sensations, as silver-chloride differs from a mere sum of its elements.

I do not think that the analogy which Dr. Broad is drawing here is a satisfactory one, even for his own purposes. For example, it is clear that this analogy might be used *against* Dr. Broad's claim that it is possible to discriminate the sensation itself in the total perceptual situation. Obviously no matter how carefully we examine the silver-chloride, we cannot detect the silver or the chlorine itself. Whichever portion of the compound we centre our attention upon, all that we can see is the compound—or a part of the compound—itself. And whatever we describe will likewise be compound or a part of it, and never the silver or the chlorine as such. Thus it is, too, I maintain, with perceptions of objects. It is a mistake to suppose that if we describe what we see in perception in neutral terms, such as 'brown patch of such and such a shape, etc.', we are thereby describing a sensation, rather than our perception of a chair.

There are, moreover, certain important respects in which the silver-chloride example differs from that of perception. We may literally take the simple elements, silver and chlorine, and combine them before our eyes in the laboratory to form the compound with its 'emergent' characteristics. Obviously, we cannot do this with sensations. Conversely, we may take the compound of silver-chloride and literally separate it into its silver and chlorine elements. But we cannot break a perception down to a mere sum of sensations. We can centre our attention on a portion of the chair we perceive, and note the colour of that portion. But this is to see a portion of an object we are perceiving; it does not mean that we are sensing a sensum. At least Dr. Broad has not yet shown this.

To be sure, we should not be able to see a chair unless our sensory apparatus was stimulated by the chair. And, of course this means that all the various separate visual qualities of the chair must somehow stimulate our eyes. But here two things must be noted. In the first place, the stimulus of light which excites the retina of our eyes does so 'all at once', and not separately. A complex stimulus affects our eyes *as* a complex stimulus, and not as a sum of separate simple qualities. Secondly, we must remember that Dr. Broad means by a sensation not a *physiological* process, but rather a *mental* awareness of a quality. Hence, regardless of what does in fact occur on the physiological level, it is still true that the only thing that occurs on the conscious *mental* level, with which alone we are concerned, is, from the very first, the perception of the chair. Dr. Broad seems to be well aware of the fact that we do not in perception *first* experience simple isolated qualities, and *then* arrive at the perception of the chair. In perceiving a chair, the very first visual experience we have is of the chair. Yet he speaks as though we first had sensations (i.e., mental awareness of simple isolated qualities), and *subsequently* arrive at the visual experience: chair. But if a visual sensation is a mental awareness, and our mental awareness is, from the start, of the chair, it is obvious that Dr. Broad must be mistaken in holding that sensations play an indispensable part in perceptual situations. They play no part at all.

In the sense in which Dr. Broad means to say it, it is not true, moreover, that there cannot be perceptual situations without sensations. What is true, I suppose, is that if we were not able to perceive each of the simple qualities which can be distinguished within our total perception of a chair, we should not be able to see them when they occur together in a chair. If we could not see the simple quality red when it occurred in isolation, then it would certainly be difficult to understand how we could perceive a complex object which numbered red among its configuration of qualities. But it does not follow from this that at the time when we are seeing a complex object, we are having the isolated kind of mental experience which can properly be called a sensation.

It is apparent, then, that what seemed to be an innocuous observation with which everyone was supposed to agree, turns out, upon examination, to be a highly debatable point. Dr. Broad has here clearly gone beyond the statement of the 'facts' of perception to introduce a notion which is in fact a part of his theory about the analysis of the facts. It suits his theory nicely to say that our perception of objects depends upon the sensing of simple qualities. These simple qualities become for him the qualities of a kind of *thing*, a sensum, which is not to be identified with physical objects, nor with any part of them. And thus he is able to generate the problem of whether or not we could possibly *know* that there are such things as physical objects, if all we are ever sensuously aware of are another kind of thing: sensa.

To conclude this discussion, I may observe that there is something innocent enough about Dr. Broad's statement that perceptual situations are 'sensuous'. Everyone would agree, certainly, that the perception of external physical objects and events is a process that occurs through the external sensory apparatus. It is a temporally immediate and causally direct process, and in these respects it certainly differs from memory, for example, in which the sensory relation to the external physical object or event is at best remote and indirect. But if this were all that Dr. Broad meant by his assertion that 'there cannot be perceptual situations without sensations', and that 'sensations play a part in perceptual situations which they do not play in any other kind of situation', it is certainly difficult to understand why he did not say so clearly and unambiguously. Mine is the sort of statement with which, I believe, everyone *would* agree. But Dr. Broad's statements are not clear. They suggest a type of analysis with which everyone certainly would not agree. In view of the results of our investigation, our caution about accepting those statements seems entirely justified.

CHAPTER II

'PHYSICAL OBJECT' AND 'OBJECTIVE CONSTITUENT'

I N the preceding chapter I examined critically Dr. Broad's presentation of what he supposes to be the facts about perceptual situations with which everyone, whatever his philosophical position, would agree. Following the ennumeration of these points, Dr. Broad states that he believes that everyone is also really agreed about 'the irreducible minimum of characteristics that a thing would have to possess in order to count as a physical object'. Having in turn enumerated these, he then goes on to inquire whether anything which possesses *all* of them is actually a 'constituent' of perceptual situations. In this chapter I want to examine what Dr. Broad has to say about the notion of 'physical object' and its connection with what he calls the 'objective constitutent' of perceptual situations.

I

Dr. Broad sets forth five marks which, he says, seem to characterize anything that we should be willing to call a 'physical object'. Briefly, these are as follows:

(i) It is conceived to be a strand of history of reasonably long duration, . . . and possessed of a characteristic unity and continuity. . . . (ii) It is conceived to be quite literally extended in space. It has some size and some shape, an inside as well as an outside, and it stands in spatial relations to other physical objects. (iii) It is conceived to persist and interact with other physical objects when no one perceives it. 'Being perceived' is regarded as something which happens from time to time to physical objects, but which is not essential to their existence, and makes no further difference to their qualities either at the time or afterwards. (iv) It is conceived to be perceptible by a number of different observers at various times. (v) It is supposed to combine a number of other qualities beside the spatio-temporal characteristics already mentioned. Some of these qualities reveal themselves in one way, others in another way; thus colour reveals itself to sight, hardness and temperature to touch, and so on.[1]

Now though Dr. Broad's fuller statement of these five characteristics provides some fruitful remarks for incidental critical analysis, I want to go on to consider his subsequent remarks, which are of more direct relevance to the main outline of the argument.

2

Having described the 'irreducible minimum of characteristics' of anything that we should be willing to call a 'physical object', Dr. Broad goes on to say:

If there be no things which have all these characteristics, there are, strictly speaking, no physical objects; and all perceptual situations are delusive. But of course there might still be things which literally possessed some of these characteristics and to which the rest could be ascribed in various more or less Pickwickian senses. In that case it would be a matter of taste whether we still said that we believed in physical objects; but it would be a matter of fact that all perceptual situations are delusive in certain respects.[2]

Now in raising this possibility, of course, Dr. Broad has in mind a subsequent development in his argument; and I shall consider this in due time. However, something may be said here by way of preliminary comment.

There is something extremely puzzling about Dr. Broad's remarks in this passage. Let us see, now. He began by outlining the characteristics of anything we should be willing to call a 'physical object'. If his outline is satisfactory, it follows that these characteristics will apply to anything we ordinarily do term a 'physical object'; and conversely, that anything which we should not be willing to designate a 'physical object' will be found, in

---

[1] *The Mind and Its Place in Nature*, pp. 145 f.
[2] *Idem*, p. 147.

fact, to lack one or more of these essential characteristics. This much is all right. But it is the suggestion that 'if there be no things which have all these characteristics, there are, strictly speaking, no physical objects', which I find so strange. Is this a plausible possibility which Dr. Broad is suggesting?

Now it must be borne in mind that the possibility which Dr. Broad is suggesting here is not that there once were objects which had all these characteristics (as one might hold that there were once dinosaurs, but there no longer are); rather he means to suggest the possibility that there are not now any such things as physical objects, and that there *never were* things which met all the defining characteristics which he has outlined. And this, I submit, is a manifestly absurd suggestion. If nothing does or ever did meet the set of requirements which Dr. Broad says characterize our notion of a physical object, the proper conclusion to be drawn from this is obviously not that there are no such things as physical objects, but rather either that he has failed to formulate this set of characteristics correctly, or else that he is applying the words he has used to formulate them in extraordinary senses. For the term 'physical object' has a perfectly good usage in English. It is a term which was devised to refer to a definite kind of object of experience—unlike, for example, the term 'unicorn'; and obviously there must be *some* things to which it is correctly applied. This seems to me to be beyond denial.

I do not think that Dr. Broad escapes this, moreover, when he allows that undoubtedly this term does apply to some experience, but that we are mistaken in what we believe about the nature of what is revealed in such experience. Consider the sort of thing we do believe about the nature of what is revealed in the kind of experience we call 'seeing a physical object'. For instance, we believe (*know!*) that physical objects are coloured, and that they have the colour they do, whatever it happens to be, regardless of whether or not we happen to be looking at them. Now some to whom it has been pointed out that the experience of colour depends upon the retina of the eye, etc., have become puzzled to the extent of wanting to say that therefore we have been in error whenever we have spoken of a physical object as being red, or yellow, or blue. But this is sheer confusion. In the first place, the fact that an individual may, for example, suffer from the kind of retinal deficiency which gives rise to the condition known as colour-blindness no more justifies the conclusion that physical objects are not themselves coloured, or that their colour is *produced* in perception, than does the fact that other individuals may have the kind of retinal deficiency which results in total blindness justify the conclusion that objects do not themselves have sensible (i.e., *capable of being perceived*) size and shape, or that these characteristics are *produced* in perception. (I shall discuss this point at greater length in a subsequent chapter.)

What those who are guilty of this confusion fail to appreciate, in the second place, is that such an expression as 'This object is red' does not *say* anything about the object that does not refer directly to what is experienced. At least, such an expression did not *say* anything when it first came into use. *Now*, of course, it does say something, in the sense that its meaning refers beyond the given experience itself. But it is important to notice the extent to which this is so. To say on any occasion subsequent to the hypothetical one in which the expression was coined, that *another* object 'is red' is to say that it has the same colour as the first object or the same colour as those objects which were indicated when the expression 'is red' was first explained to us in our childhoods, ostensively, as it obviously must have been.

To be sure, the matter is somewhat more complex than this. We mean to say that not only does the particular object have the same colour as did the defining one, but that it has it *in the same way*. That is, we are aware that often an object will only *appear* to have a certain colour because it is being illuminated by light of that colour, or because it is covered with a bit of coloured cellophane paper, etc.; and when we say of a given object that it 'is red', generally, I believe, we mean to say that it is red in the normal way, and that its redness is not due to such extraordinary factors.

But now, supposing that such expressions as 'This table is red' do mean both of these things, what is it that anyone who denies that such propositions (which, it may be noted, entail the further proposition that 'physical objects are coloured') are ever really true is doing? Is he denying that the object does have the same colour as the defining one? We can show him that it compares favourably. Perhaps he is denying that it has *exactly* the same colour? Then we must explain to him that we don't necessarily mean '*exactly* the same colour' when we make such statements. On the other hand, is he claiming that this object is not coloured *in the same way* as in the defining case? But this is a matter which can be settled empirically.

If these matters be clarified, then, what is it that one is denying when he denies the literal truth of such expressions as 'This table is red', or 'Physical objects are coloured'? Obviously there is nothing relevant which he could be denying. Hence, I conclude that anyone who holds that 'there are, strictly speaking, no physical objects', on the ground that nothing accurately fulfils the characteristic of literally 'being coloured', which is one of the requirements specified for 'being a physical object', is either shockingly unobservant, or else he is failing to understand how we employ such phrases as 'is red', 'is blue', 'is coloured'. And the same argument would apply, *mutatis mutandis*, for any of the other characteristics which we ordinarily predicate of anything we call a 'physical object'.

Dr. Broad is thus entertaining a notion which is patently absurd, when he suggests that the senses in which the things which we call 'physical objects' have the properties which we ordinarily ascribe to them may be *Pickwickian*. The sense of a term or of an expression in a given context can properly be termed Pickwickian only if that term or expression is there used in a special or esoteric sense—only, that is, if that term or expression is borrowed from another, essentially different and more fundamental usage. But this is clearly not the case with the ordinary language we employ in talking about physical objects and their qualities and characteristics. Quite on the contrary, in such contexts we employ these words in their *proper* senses; for it was in the context of propositions about those items of sense-experience which we ordinarily call physical objects that such fundamental terms were originally denotatively defined. Hence, the ordinary assertions we make about physical objects and their qualities are true (or, as the case may sometimes be, false) *literally*. And I think that this is so patently true that we can say beforehand that any arguments which Dr. Broad might adduce to the contrary must be, *ipso facto*, sophistical.

3

Now sentences like 'I see a chair' or 'I hear a bell', which are typical linguistic expressions for perceptual situations, Dr. Broad says, invariably suggest a certain mode of analysis for the perceptual situation. This analysis is comprised of me and the physical object whose name appears in the phrase, related by an asymmetrical two-term relation which is indicated by the verb. And this, he observes, suggests that the admitted existence of the situation guarantees the existence of me and of the physical object. 'How far', asks Dr. Broad, 'can this simple-minded view be maintained?'[1]

In philosophy it is equally silly to be a slave to common speech or to neglect it. When we remember that it represents the analyses made unconsciously for practical ends by our prehistoric ancestors we shall not be inclined to treat it as an oracle. When we remember that they were probably no greater fools than we are, we shall recognize that it is likely to accord at any rate with the more obvious facts, and that it will be wise to take it as our starting-point and to work from it. It is plausible to suppose that the perceptual situation which language describes by the phrase 'I see a chair' does contain two outstanding constituents related by an asymmetrical two-term relation. But it is quite another question whether these two constituents can possibly be what is commonly understood by 'me' and by 'chair'.[2]

With respect to these remarks, I think that the comments contained in the preceding section apply here with equal force. But I think that the following may also be said. In the first place, expressions like 'I see a chair', etc., do indeed suggest the sort of analysis which Dr. Broad describes, into subject and object. It is not quite clear, however, just what he means when he adds that such an analysis in turn suggests that the admitted existence of the situation guarantees the existence of 'me' and of the physical object. If Dr. Broad means by the 'situation' a case where I *truly* say that I see a chair, and am not the victim of either an illusion or of an hallucination, in the usual sense in which some persons are occasionally so victimized, then I should say that the 'existence of the situation' necessarily guaranteed the existence of 'me' and of the physical object. On the other hand, if he means by the 'situation' merely a visual experience, and there is some doubt as to whether the experience is veridical or hallucinatory, then, of course, the existence of such a situation would obviously not guarantee the existence of the physical object (though it would,

[1] *Idem*, p. 148.
[2] *Ibid*.

to be sure, guarantee the existence of whoever was the subject whose experience it was). I do not suppose that anyone, no matter how 'simple-minded', is not aware of the fact that occasionally one thinks he sees an object, and subsequently learns that he was mistaken in so thinking, or in thinking that the object was of the sort he originally took it to be.

But now what does Dr. Broad mean when he says that in philosophy it is equally silly to be a slave to common speech or to neglect it? I can see, for example, that it would be silly to be misled by the fact that we speak of 'having an illusion', into maintaining that when one 'has' an illusion there is a *thing* which he *has*, in the same sense that there is when he has a penny; or to be misled by the fact that we say 'I see an after-image', into supposing that some*thing* corresponds to the object term ('after-image'), just as a thing does correspond to the term 'penny' in the superficially similar expression 'I see a penny'. On the other hand, the fact that we alternatively speak of 'having' an after-image, whereas we cannot with the same meaning substitute 'having' for 'seeing' in the sentence 'I see a penny', gives us a clue to the difference between the two situations. Being a 'slave to common speech' would perhaps consist of dogmatically arguing exclusively from similarity of expression to similarity of situation, without taking account of differences in meaning. 'Neglecting common speech' would perhaps consist in disregarding the evidences of difference offered to analysis by differences in usage, as in the case above.

This, however, is obviously not what Dr. Broad has in mind when he says that common speech represents the 'analyses made unconsciously for practical ends by our prehistoric ancestors'. But what, then, does he mean? Philology gives us examples of languages which differ somewhat in their construction as well as in vocabulary. But the sensory experiences of all men are basically the same. Our ancestors picked up objects, handled them, exchanged them, etc. And they also perceived them and described them. They saw that objects differ in size, shape, colour, and so forth. But the fact that they coined words and developed a language testifies to the fact that they also recognized that there were similarities between objects and their behaviour and the ways in which they could be dealt with. These similarities or repetitive aspects of experience were fixed in the common nouns, adjectives, verbs, adverbs, and prepositions of our language. Our prehistoric ancestors undoubtedly recognized, for example, the similarity between picking up a stick and picking up a stone, and they abstracted the common activity and instigated the convention of designating it by the expression 'picking up', or its equivalent in whatever sounds they employed. Similarly, a name arose to refer to the experience of being visually aware of, which we call 'seeing'. In time language became formalized, with a syntax and an extensive vocabulary to refer to the various discernible differences and similarities within experience, in all their subtlety and complexity.

These differences and similarities were no doubt distinguished and given special designations in language on the basis of practical ends; but this is not to say that they did not reflect perceivable aspects of experience itself. It is conceivable, for example, that a given language might lack expressions for 'on', 'under', etc., perhaps subsuming them all under a single term, such as 'by'. But still, words like 'on' and 'under' do express differences which can be discerned, regardless of the historical fact that our ancestors obviously found it useful to distinguish them by different specific word-designations. Similarly, there is no end to the number of different words we can coin to designate the subtle differences between various instances of the sort of relationship we now designate as simply 'under'. We could employ a special word for the situation in which an object is one inch below another, another special word for situations in which an object is two inches below another, and so on. And as a matter of fact, some languages differ from English in precisely this sort of way. But English is just as serviceable, because we can indicate these differences by different combinations of words. Be all this as it may, however, the fact remains that these designations are not purely whimsical and arbitrary. They designate observable aspects of experience.

It seems to me, then, that all that our ancestors were responsible for was the fixation of useful distinctions and similarities in our common experience by special names which have come down to us. Had they failed to provide a workable mode of communication for us, then in time we would have perfected one, more or less along the lines of our present language system, by adding the distinctions of syntax and vocabulary for which we have need, even though our ancestors had been able to get along without them. This is the only sense in which I can understand what Dr. Broad means by the 'analyses' which our prehistoric ancestors made for us in their common speech. The usefulness of the (still growing) language which we have inherited from them testifies to the correctness or, better, the adequacy of the 'analyses' which they 'unconsciously made'—i.e., the distinctions of syntax and vocabulary. The expression 'I see a chair' states a proposition which is sometimes, in fact very often, true in precisely the sense in which its users intend. Our success in communicating in this fashion is pragmatic proof of this. If the two constituents which make up the situation expressed by the proposition 'I see a chair' were not what is commonly understood by 'me' and by 'chair', as Dr. Broad suggests, it is certainly incomprehensible how it is that we communicate successfully in this way, using these words.

I want to consider, nevertheless, the grounds on which Dr. Broad contends that a perceptual situation, such as that indicated by the expression 'I see a chair', does not *contain as constituents* what is commonly understood by 'me' and by 'chair'. Now Dr. Broad distinguishes between what he calls the '*objective* constituent' of the perceptual situation, and what he calls the '*subjective* constituent'. The latter involves, on his analysis, 'the mass of bodily feeling together with the "mnemic consequences' of the apprehension of the sensum'. In the preceding chapter (Section 4) I had occasion to consider something of what Dr. Broad has to say about the 'subjective constituent' in connection with the distinction which he makes between sensation and perception. In the present analysis I am concerned solely with what he terms the '*objective* constituent'.

Dr. Broad has said that the typical linguistic expression for the perceptual situation 'I see a chair' suggests a certain mode of analysis for the perceptual situation. However, he goes on to say: 'Even if we had never had any reason to believe that some perceptual situations are delusive, this extremely simple-minded analysis would need to be modified considerably.'[1] In support of this statement he offers three arguments, which I propose to consider in turn.

(*a*) It would be admitted that in any one perceptual situation I am never aware of the *whole* of the surface of a physical object, in the

[1] *Idem*, pp. 148 f.

sense in which I seem to be aware of a part of it. Nobody who was looking at a bell would seriously maintain that, at a given moment, he is aware of the far side and the inside of the bell, in the same sense in which he would claim to be aware of a certain part of the outside which is facing him at the time. And by a 'bell' we certainly mean something which has a closed surface with an inside as well as an outside, and not merely a patch with indefinite boundaries. Thus the most we could say is: 'The perceptual situation contains as a constituent something which is in fact part of the surface of a bell.'[1]

Now the peculiar thing about what Dr. Broad is saying here, is that though so much of it is true, there is something not quite right about what he thinks it amounts to, and about the conclusion he consequently wants to draw. It is true, for example, that when I look at a bell, at any one moment I can see only a part of its surface. And it is also true that by a 'bell' we mean 'something which has a closed surface with an inside as well as an outside, and not merely a patch with indefinite boundaries'. But is it true that the most we could say is: 'The perceptual situation contains as a constituent something which is in fact part of the surface of a bell'?

Suppose we were to ask: 'Do you see that building?' Would it be quite appropriate to reply: 'No, I don't. I only see the part of its surface facing me'? This would be taken as a poor attempt at humour, to which the proper reply would be something like: 'But of course! How else did you expect to see it?' For though it is true that I can see only the part of its surface facing me, it isn't true that I don't see the building; though I don't see *all* of the building, it is still true that I see the building. That is what 'seeing a building' is like; that is what the expression *means*. If our eyes were constructed differently, say like our arms, we would be able to surround objects with them and see all of their surfaces at once. But 'seeing an object' means the sort of thing that occurs when we look at an object before us, with the kind of eyes we do have.

If one is going to make the sort of objection Dr. Broad does, one might as well say that we can never feel an object, because all we touch is a small portion of its surface; or that we can never taste a stick of peppermint candy, because all we touch with our tongues is a portion of its surface; or that we can't place a book on a table, because the book would occupy only a small portion of

[1] *Idem*, p. 149.

the upper surface of the table; or that I am not sitting on a chair, because I am not sitting all over it. To this sort of absurd objection the only reply, if, indeed, it deserves one, is: '*Of course* we are tasting the candy, feeling the object, seeing the building, etc. What else did you think doing these things was like? Who ever heard of seeing both the outside and the inside of a solid, opaque object, simultaneously!'

It is perfectly true that by a 'bell' we mean 'something which has a closed surface with an inside as well as an outside, and not merely a patch with indefinite boundaries'. But in the first place, 'seeing a bell' does not mean simultaneously seeing *all* of its surface, its inside and its outside, etc. And in the second place, when we see or touch a bell, we *are* seeing or touching something which has all these characteristics. It is true, but trivial, to point out that at any one moment we are seeing or touching only a part of the surface of something which has all these characteristics. From the fact that we are seeing or touching only a part of its surface, it does not follow that we are not seeing or touching the object; nor that the object doesn't have all these characteristics. Of course, on the other hand, it does not follow from the fact that we are sensuously aware of only a part of its surface at a given moment, that the object does have all these characteristics. The object might be only a cast of a half of a bell. But if it does have all these characteristics, then it *is* a bell, and the matter is settled.

What, then, is Dr. Broad saying when he concludes that the most we could say is that 'The perceptual situation contains as a constituent something which is in fact part of the surface of a bell'? Let us consider again just what is meant by a 'perceptual situation' and by a 'constituent' of such a situation. Dr. Broad, it will be recalled, declared that he would call such situations as are 'naturally indicated by phrases like "I am seeing a chair" or "I am hearing a bell" by the name of "Perceptual Situations"'.[1] What sort of situations *are* naturally indicated by such phrases? The proper answer, it seems to me, is obviously: those in which there is a chair, or a ringing bell, and the speaker is visually or auditorily aware of them. Such situations, as Dr. Broad has suggested, are commonly considered as having two outstanding 'constituents', related by an asymmetrical two-term relation.

[1] *Idem*, p. 141. Cf. *supra*, Ch. I, Sec. 2.

And in the case of 'I see a chair,' these are the person who sees and the chair. But now, if this is what is meant by a 'perceptual situation' and by a 'constituent', then Dr. Broad is certainly wrong in saying that the most that we could say is that the perceptual 'I see a bell' contains as a constituent something which is in fact only part of the surface of a bell. We can, of course, say this; but we can also say that it contains as a constituent the whole bell (provided, naturally, that the situation expressed by the words 'I see a bell' is not delusive, in the usual sense).

Of course, if Dr. Broad wants to limit the 'perceptual situation' so as to include as the 'objective constituent' only that part of the bell which is directly visible at any one moment, why then naturally that is 'the most we could say'. But if he does mean to delimit it so, then we may say, in the first place, that he does not mean by 'perceptual situations' such situations as are *naturally* and ordinarily indicated by phrases like 'I am seeing a bell', etc. For situations naturally expressed in this manner are those, as I have pointed out, which involve a bell and someone who sees them. And in the second place, Dr. Broad is mistaken in holding that the 'naïve analysis' of the situation must be modified; for it is clear that he does not mean the same thing by 'perceptual situation' as those who offer the 'naïve analysis' mean. If the latter understood by this phrase what Dr. Broad intends, they would not, I am certain, disagree with what is obviously a truism.

There is still another objection which may be urged against the sort of language which Dr. Broad claims is more adequate and correct than ordinary speech. Suppose the crack in the Liberty Bell in Philadelphia were to progress so that the bell were split into pieces. And suppose that these pieces were then sent to various museums in the country. Then a visitor who was examining one of the pieces might naturally say: 'I am seeing only a part of the surface of a bell'—i.e., not a whole bell. Now it is only of such a perceptual situation that the most we could say, ordinarily, is that it contained as a constituent something which is in fact only part of the surface of a bell. As a matter of fact, to get it exactly right, the piece that the speaker was seeing would have to be only a surface chip of the bell, and not a piece which included an entire thickness of the wall of the original bell. Then, and only then, would it be natural and proper to say: 'I am seeing only a part of the surface of a bell.' But in any case, these words are here being used in a sense in which it would not be proper or natural to use them if one were looking at the Liberty Bell in its present, whole, condition.

5

Let us see now what we can do with the similar limitation with regard to *duration* which Dr. Broad says must be put upon the 'naïve analysis' of the perceptual situation. He writes:

(*b*) A similar limitation with regard to time must be put on the naïve analysis of the perceptual situation. By a 'bell' we mean something of considerable duration; something which certainly may, and almost certainly does, stretch out in time beyond the limits of the perceptual situation in which I am aware of it. Now no one would maintain that the parts of the history of the bell which come before the beginning and after the end of a certain perceptual situation are 'given' to him in that perceptual situation in the same sense in which the contemporary slice of the bell's history is 'given'. Thus we have no right to say that the situation described by the phrase 'I am seeing the bell' contains the *bell* as a constituent; at most we can say that it contains as a constituent a short event which is in fact a slice of a longer strand of history, and that this longer strand is the history of a certain bell.[1]

Here again, if I understand him aright, Dr. Broad is quite correct in what he says we mean by a 'bell'. A bell *is* 'something which certainly may, and almost certainly does, stretch out in time beyond the limits of the perceptual situation in which I am aware of it'. He is also right when he says that 'no one would maintain that the parts of the history of the bell which came before the beginning and after the end of a certain perceptual situation are "given" to him in that perceptual situation in the same sense in which the contemporary slice of the bell's history is "given"'. 'Parts of the history of the bell' and 'slice of the bell's history' is highly figurative language, to be sure; but it seems clear what Dr. Broad has in mind here. Obviously one doesn't see the bell *before* he *begins* to see it, nor *after* he *ceases* to see it. Dr. Broad certainly has us here! But now what are we to say concerning his conclusion that 'we have no right to say that the situation described by the phrase "I am seeing the bell" contains the *bell* as a constituent;'

[1] *Idem*, p. 149.

and that 'at most we can say that it contains as a constituent a short event which is in fact a slice of a longer strand of history, and that this longer strand is the history of a certain bell'?

Now in the case of the first qualification which Dr. Broad advanced, the fact that when we see an object we see only a portion of its surface at any given moment, there was a certain plausibility to his insistence that only a part of the surface of the bell was a constituent of the perceptual situation. This plausibility stemmed, to be sure, from his delimitation of the 'perceptual situation' to include only that part of the bell which is actually visible to a given observer at any moment. But despite the fact that there is good reason to argue the artificiality of such a delimitation, Dr. Broad's conclusion at least followed from his definition, in that case. With respect to the qualification based on the present argument involving duration, however, I can see no basis at all for the conclusion that the object itself could not be a constituent of a perceptual situation. His premise about duration, as I have shown, comes to nothing more than the obvious truism that we do not see an object before or after we see it. And it simply does not follow at all from the fact that we do not see an object before or after we see it, that the object is not a constituent of the situation in which we do see it.

Dr. Broad seems to be supposing, without warrant, that what is usually true of physical objects must be true of the situations in which they are perceived, if it is to be possible to hold that they are constituents of the situations in which they are perceived. Now it is usually true, of course, that objects have an existence that is longer in duration than the periods during which they are perceived by a given individual. But Dr. Broad is mistaken in supposing that the duration of the perception must be co-extensive with that of the object, in order for one to be able to say, correctly: 'I see a bell'. Even if someone were to claim that the *whole* bell was literally a constituent of this perceptual situation, the fact that the duration of the existence of the bell extended beyond the temporal limits of the perceptual situation described in this way would obviously not be good reason for denying the literal truth of this proposition. For a 'whole' bell does not mean the whole *history* of a bell. Consider the following, moreover. All that Dr. Broad has said is that by a 'bell' we mean something which may and usually does 'stretch out in time' beyond the limits of the perceptual situation in which we are aware of it. And I think this may very easily be granted. But now, when I look, at some given time, at the Liberty Bell in Philadelphia, is it not true that I am seeing something of which it is true that it 'stretches out in time' beyond the limits of the perceptual situation in which I am aware of it? The proud citizens of Philadelphia would assure me that it most certainly is. The point is simply this: 'seeing something which (also) existed before I see it, and which will continue to exist after I see it' does not mean 'seeing it before and after I see it'. It is perfectly correct to say, in the appropriate situation, that 'I see a bell'. And when I say this, and it is true in the ordinary sense, then, at least so far as the present argument is concerned, the whole bell, which is a physical object, is a constituent of the situation.

What, then, is the point of this strange talk about 'slices of history', 'longer strands of history', 'short events', etc.? So far as I can see, its purpose seems to be to avoid the use of the terms 'physical object', 'bell', etc., which would, so to speak, obviously 'give the show away'. But Dr. Broad is, of course, mistaken, if he supposes that such terms as 'slice', 'strand', 'history', 'events', etc., can be understood apart from the meaning of such terms as 'physical object' and 'bell'. And it is also clear that if the former are to convey any meaning, they must do so in their familiar senses; and these are, of course, derived from the context of what is ordinarily understood by the term 'physical objects'.

Finally, it is again obvious that it is purely a verbal disagreement which Dr. Broad is maintaining against the 'naïve analysis' of common sense. For he surely is not maintaining anything with which anyone disagrees, when he insists that objects exist before and after the period during which we may happen to perceive them, and that we cannot see them before we begin to see them, nor after we cease to see them. If someone were to query, as I was looking at the Liberty Bell: 'Do you see the bell?' And I were to reply that I didn't, and then cite Dr. Broad's argument in defence, that someone would very likely retort that I knew very well what the question meant, and that I had simply answered incorrectly. And, of course, he would be right. The situation that existed then was precisely that which is *meant* by the expression 'I see a bell'. To hold that it isn't, or that the 'whole' bell wasn't literally a constituent of that situation, for the reason that

Dr. Broad gives, is simply to legislate some new and unusual meanings for some very common expressions.

6

Similar criticisms apply to Dr. Broad's third objection to what he calls the 'naïve analysis' of perceptual situations:

(*c*) It would be admitted by every one that a bell is something more than a coloured surface, more than a cold hard surface, and so on. Now, so long as I merely look at a bell, its colour only is revealed to me; its temperature or hardness are certainly not revealed in the same sense at that time. Similarly, when I merely touch the bell, only its temperature and hardness are revealed to me; its colour is certainly not revealed to me in the same sense at that time. Once again then I have no right to say that the *bell* is a constituent of either of these perceptual situations. At most I may say there is a constituent which displays certain qualities, and that this same constituent has in fact other qualities which would be displayed under other conditions.[1]

Once more Dr. Broad begins with a perfectly true statement. A bell certainly is something more than a coloured surface, more than a cold, hard surface, and so on. For there are coloured, cold hard surfaces which are not the surfaces of bells. He is also right when he says that so long as he merely looks at a bell, only its colour (i.e., only its immediately visible characteristics) is revealed to him; its temperature or its hardness are certainly not revealed to him at the same time in the same sense. Here is another of Dr. Broad's truistic statements. When you merely look at something (i.e., don't also feel it, taste it, etc.), why of course you can't feel its hardness and coldness, or taste its bitterness. And when you only touch it, and don't also see it, why, then, of course you don't see its colour. But again Dr. Broad draws a conclusion whose relevance to the evidence he offers for it is very difficult to see.

From the fact that when you look at an object, a bell, for instance, and don't also touch it, you perceive only its visual qualities and not its tactual qualities, it does not seem to me to follow that you are not entitled to say 'I see a bell'. For, granted that a bell can be described in all the sense-modalities, it still does not follow that because you happen to be sensing it in only

[1] *Idem*, pp. 149 f.

74

one these modalities, that of sight, for instance, you are not, therefore, seeing a bell. The proper reply to Dr. Broad's objection should be: 'Did you expect to feel it when you only looked at it? What's so strange about the fact that you don't feel it when you only look at it, that should cause you to decide that you were wrong in saying "I see a bell" on those occasions when you did say this? Have you ever, or at least very often, found that your assertion was incorrect? Did you say this, and think this, and then find when you tried to feel it or hear it that what you had seen was not a bell after all, but something else? I don't suppose that this has happened to you often enough to make you insist that we change our mode of speaking so drastically. Why, then, should it be wrong to say, as we ordinarily do, that what we see is a bell, or at least part of the surface of a bell? Of course a bell can be perceived through the other senses. But isn't it possible only to look at a bell? A physical object, as you say, has various other qualities besides those which can be seen; but doesn't the bell which you are looking at also have these characteristics? Feel it, taste it, smell it, hear it; see for yourself if it doesn't! You are not, it is true, at the moment perceiving these other qualities; but what of it? As we have already agreed, and you have not yet, at any rate, contradicted this: physical objects persist and interact with other physical objects when no one perceives them. "Being perceived" is not essential to their existence, and hence it is not essential to those other physical characteristics which are capable of being experienced qualitatively, though they do not at the moment happen to be.'

Finally, I want to call attention to the possibility of confusing what Dr. Broad is here arguing with another and quite different argument. He is not here arguing merely that when one only looks, that is, when one is merely having a visual experience, he can't be sure that the 'object' has these other characteristics—i.e., that he is really seeing an object, and not merely having an hallucination. If to 'be sure' means to have direct experiential evidence, then it is, of course, true that when one only looks, he can't be sure. But if this were all that Professor Broad is arguing, then he would have to allow that afterwards, when one had verified the accuracy of his visual experience by means of his other senses, and by the confirmation of other observers, one could say with justification: 'I see a bell', or at least: 'I was seeing a bell'. Anyone who had already made sure in this way could then *know* that he was right in saying 'I see a bell', and wouldn't have to limit himself to Dr. Broad's narrow statement. But it is evident that this is not the kind of argument that Dr. Broad is advancing. The one he is advancing does not have this kind of justification. And it cannot be met in this empirical way. It is a verbal issue.

7

In view of the considerations which I have advanced against Dr. Broad's three progressively more dubious arguments, I feel that there is ample ground, then, for refusing to concede his conclusion that:

Thus we are forced to modify the first naïve analysis of 'I see a bell' at least in the following respects: We cannot hold that this situation literally contains the bell itself as a constituent. The most we can say is that the situation contains me and *something* related by an asymmetrical two-term relation; that this something is in fact a part of a larger surface, and is also a short slice of a longer strand of history; that it has in fact other qualities beside those which are sensuously revealed to me in this situation; and that this spatially larger and temporally longer whole, with the qualities which are not revealed sensuously in this situation, is a certain bell. This whole is the epistemological object of the situation expressed by the phrase 'I am seeing the bell'. And, even if it be granted that there is an ontological object which corresponds accurately to the epistemological object, we cannot admit that *it* is bodily a constituent of the situation. The most we can grant is that a small spatio-temporal fragment of the ontological object is literally a constituent of the situation, and that a small selection of the qualities of this fragment is sensuously revealed in the situation.[1]

So far as the three arguments we have discussed are concerned, it is clear that all that Dr. Broad has succeeded in showing is the somewhat obvious set of facts that we can be sensibly aware of only a part of the surface of a physical object at any moment, that we do not see an object during the time we are not seeing it, and that when we only *see* it, we do not also feel it, taste it, smell it, etc. But now he refers to the 'spatially larger and temporally longer whole, with the qualities which are not revealed sensuously in this situation', as a certain bell, which is the epistemological

[1] *Idem*, p. 150.

object of the situation expressed by the phrase 'I am seeing the bell'. We recall that in his statement of the facts' Dr. Broad gave us to understand that he means by an 'epistemological object' the claim to be in cognitive contact with something other than ourselves and our states. Now granting the set of propositions which Dr. Broad has advanced concerning the extent to which we are sensuously aware of the bell in such a situation as is naturally indicated by the expression 'I am seeing a bell', I fail to see that Dr. Broad has shown that this claim is false. No one who claims to see a bell claims to have more *sensory* contact with it than a visual perception of a part of its surface. But he does claim to be in cognitive contact with something which has all the characteristics of the kind of physical object that a bell is. And people are very often correct when they make this claim. For if they see a part of the surface of a bell, then they are seeing a part of something which does have all these characteristics. In the sense in which the statement is intended, moreover, they are perfectly correct when they claim that they are seeing a bell. For just as seeing a tree does not mean seeing its roots and the sap in its veins at the same time as one is seeing its bark-covered surface and leaves, so seeing a bell does not mean being sensorily aware of all of the qualities of every portion of it at the same time. It means being in visual sensory contact with a physical object which does have all of these characteristics. And being in visual sensory contact with something which does have all of these characteristics means being in sensory contact with that part of the object which is directly visible from a given place at a given time.

If Dr. Broad means to use the term 'perceptual situation' to refer to such situations as are naturally indicated by phrases like 'I am seeing a chair', etc., as he said at the outset, and if he means by the 'objective constituent' of such situations that which is seen when the situation is veridical, then his remarks in the passage just quoted strike me as being exceedingly strange. Consider: suppose I were to carry a bell into the room and place it before someone so that he might look at it. Here I would be arranging a situation whose constituents were a perceiving individual and a bell. It seems to me that when the individual looked at the bell, we would have a situation which might very naturally be called a 'perceptual situation'. But then, isn't the bell literally and bodily a part of this situation whose geographical boundaries would include at least the bell and the observer? How seriously can we take the argument that inasmuch as I hadn't tasted, smelled and heard the bell as well as looked at it, and inasmuch as I had held it by only a part of its surface, and inasmuch as I hadn't done any of these things for anything but a relatively brief span of the bell's history, therefore I hadn't carried a bell into the room at all, but only a small spatio-temporal fragment of a bell—and at that, only a small selection of the qualities of that fragment? Such a position leads to many absurd difficulties.

Supposing that we accept Dr. Broad's delimitation of what he will call the 'perceptual situation' as being a geographical one, including only the directly visible portion of the bell, what are we to say about the *unperceived* qualities of that portion? Can we say that what we *see* in the perceptual situation, the objective constituent, is only a selection of visual qualities? A visual quality is not itself an object; it characterizes the way objects look. We don't look at qualities, but rather at objects. The qualitative experiences which objects produce when they are perceived through the various sense organs are what the various sense-quality terms like 'red', 'warm', etc., describe—though this is not incompatible, as I have shown, with statements like 'This object is red', 'This object is warm', etc.

Dr. Broad is quite correct, of course, when he says that what we mean by a bell is something which can not only be seen, but can be felt and heard as well. But we do not mean that it is something which *is* being seen, felt, and heard at all times. When I carry a bell into the room I am carrying something which *can* be seen and heard as well as felt, even though at the moment I am carrying it I may not be looking at it or hearing it. In order to set up the perceptual situation so that someone may see a part of the surface of the bell, I cannot carry into the room just the colour of that portion of the bell and set it before him. There is no sense to this proposition. How can I geographically mark off the visible portion of the bell's surface from the touchable portion of it?

Let us even suppose that this made sense. In setting up the perceptual situation which would evoke the expression 'I see a bell' from the observer, I may not look at the bell at all, but may only touch a part of its surface in carrying it into the room. In that case, according to what Dr. Broad seems to be arguing, I could not properly say that the constituent of the combined perceptual and carrying situation was a bell, but only that it was a small, spatio-temporal, single-quality slice of a longer strand of history. But now, when I place this impoverished substitute for a material object before an observer, he *sees* it. How could this be if I carried only a tactual quality into the room? Apparently I must have carried the visual qualities of that portion of the surface of the bell which I touched into the room along with its tactual qualities! But see, now: his visual perception includes a larger portion of the surface of the bell than I actually perceived in carrying it into the room, for I merely held it with my fingers. Then I must have carried more of its surface into the room than I thought I had? Again, I carried it for only a relatively short period of its history, and then set it down. But the observer is seeing it at a later date; so apparently I was not carrying and perceiving only a 'short strand of history', but something with a continuing existence. Finally, the observer walks around the object and examines it all over with all his senses, and reports that it feels cold, gives off a loud clear tone when struck, has a metallic taste, and so forth and so on. Now how could he do all this if it were not the whole bell which I had literally and bodily carried into the room and set before him?

It is precisely these characteristics of such situations that the naïve realist has in mind when he chooses to speak in terms of 'seeing a bell', even though he knows as well as Dr. Broad that at any given moment he sees only a portion of its surface, and may not at that moment be also feeling it and hearing it and tasting it. He means that the whole bell is a constituent of his perceptual situation in the sense in which it would not be if I were merely to exhibit a fragment of a bell, or to project an image of a bell upon a cloud.

8

It is impossible to suppose with any conviction that Dr. Broad is not aware of the difficulties advanced in the preceding section. The answer to this puzzle, I suspect, is to be found in what Dr. Broad actually means by a 'perceptual situation'. His statement that 'I will call such situations as are naturally indicated by phrases like "I am seeing a chair" or "I am hearing a bell" by the name of "Perceptual Situations",' turns out to be very misleading. The type of situation that is naturally indicated by such expressions is one in which there is a physical object of a certain sort, and the person speaking is perceiving it. While it is not natural to delimit such situations to include only the sensuously revealed portion of the physical object, such a delimitation would at least approximate what is 'naturally indicated' by such expressions. But it has become apparent that what Dr. Broad does mean by a 'perceptual situation' does not even approximate what would be naturally indicated by such expressions as he offers. What, then, does he mean?

It will be recalled that in the statement of the 'facts' of perception with which everyone was supposed to agree, regardless of the analysis he might subsequently prefer, Dr. Broad made it clear that he proposed to employ the term 'perceptual situation' in such a way that both veridical and hallucinatory experiences would qualify. He proposed to employ the term to refer only to that much of the two situations, 'I see a pink rat' (veridical), and 'I see a pink rat' (hallucinatory), as they would have in common (if there were such a thing as an actual pink rat). He suggested that he would refer to this common element of the two situations by means of the statements: 'There is a perceptual situation of the visual kind of which I am subject. This has such and such an epistemological object.' To allow for the difference between the two, he offered the further statement: 'And there is a physical object corresponding to this epistemological object', expressing a claim which would in the first case, but not in the second, be said to be 'met by the physical world'. Now it might be thought that these statements are innocent enough, and that we ought to indulge a philosopher in what is ostensibly a matter of verbal usage. But I want to show how in offering what appears to be merely a statement of the facts and of how he proposes to use terms, and not an analysis of perception from a particular bias, Dr. Broad is actually stacking the cards in such a way as to enhance his argument in the point at issue here.

In Section 2 of the preceding chapter, I commented on the ambiguity of the distinction which Dr. Broad makes between 'epistemological object' and the 'corresponding ontological object'. The difference between perceptual situations, such as 'I see a rat', and non-perceptual situations, such as 'I feel cross', he holds, is that in the former there is the 'claim to be in cognitive contact with some*thing* other than ourselves and our states', while in the latter no such claim is involved. This claim, he maintains, is just as obvious in those perceptual situations which are commonly believed to be delusive as in those which are commonly believed to be veridical. Dr. Broad then goes on to say that he will express the difference between veridical and delusive perceptual situations on the one hand, and the non-perceptual situation on the other, by saying that the first kind does and the second kind does not have an epistemological object. Thus, Dr. Broad's original statement of what the veridical and the delusive perceptual situations have in common, denoted by the term 'epistemological object', was that they both involve a common *claim*. But this similarity in claims, as I pointed out there, is misleadingly expressed by Dr. Broad as though veridical and delusive perceptual situations had some*thing* in common beside this claim, namely an 'epistemological *object*'. This confusion, I warned, would be the source of later difficulty.

If now we bear in mind that Dr. Broad means by a visual perceptual situation a situation involving a perceiver and something like an hallucinatory visual image, which both an hallucination and a veridical perception are supposed to have in common, it is readily understandable how he could maintain that the objective constituent of a perceptual situation is only a set of qualities in a single sense modality. For visual images, of course, do involve only the qualities of sight. And the same would hold true, *mutatis mutandis*, for hallucinatory experiences in the other modalities. But here two objections may be registered.

In the first place, we must remember that Dr. Broad was claiming to state the facts in a manner with which everyone could agree. And I cannot agree that the proper analysis of veridical and hallucinatory situations of the visual kind involves seeing images, as though both situations were hallucinatory, only the veridical involved an external physical object as well. This is just the point which I want to debate in some detail. I want to argue that we don't see physical objects via 'images' (which become for Dr. Broad the kind of objects he calls 'sensa'), as though these were intervening films. I want to argue that what we see in veridical perception are objects themselves; and that the 'image' in veridical perception is not *what we see*, but is the seeing itself, the 'look' of physical objects.

81

But now, in the second place, if this is indeed what Dr. Broad means by a 'perceptual situation', then while it is understandable how he could say what he does about the characteristics of the 'objective constituent' of such a situation, it gives rise to the greater puzzle as to why he went to the pains he did to argue that the whole physical object is not literally and bodily a constituent. Though he might object to the artificial and highly debatable manner in which Dr. Broad proposes to employ the term 'perceptual situation', the most naïve of realists would hardly deny that what Dr. Broad maintains follows from his definition. The naïve realist might deny that it was what *he* meant by a 'perceptual situation' when he held that the physical object was literally and bodily a constituent of it; and hence he might deny that Dr. Broad had shown him to be wrong. But it is obvious from the outset that not even a portion of the surface of a physical object is literally and bodily a constituent of a sensory image.

CHAPTER III

THE 'EXTERNAL REFERENCE' OF PERCEPTION

HAVING argued that perceptual situations do not and could not contain as a constituent anything that could properly be denoted by the term physical object', Dr. Broad goes on to conclude that thus the existence of the kind of situation denoted, for example, by a phrase like 'I see the bell', does not suffice to guarantee the existence of the physical object denoted by the phrase 'the bell'. Nevertheless, perceptual experiences do have an 'external reference'. Dr. Broad puts it this way:

It is plain . . . that there is involved in every perceptual situation another factor beside me and a certain spatio-temporally extended particular. This is the conviction that this particular something is not isolated and self-subsistent, and is not completely revealed in all its qualities; but that it is spatio-temporally a part of a larger whole of a certain characteristic kind, viz., a certain physical object, and that this whole has other qualities beside those which are sensuously manifested in the perceptual situation.

Let us call the constituent about which we believe these propositions 'the objective constituent of the perceptual situation'. And let us call this conviction which we have about the objective constituent 'the external reference of the situation'. I give it this name because it clearly points spatially, temporally, and qualitatively, beyond the situation and what is contained and sensuously manifested in it.[1]

In this chapter I want to examine what Dr. Broad says about the external reference of perceptual situations. He begins his analysis by arguing that we neither do, nor could we, *infer* 'from

[1] *The Mind and Its Place in Nature*, p. 151.

the mere presence of an objective constituent, which sensuously manifests such and such qualities, that this constituent is part of a larger spatio-temporal whole which is not a constituent of the situation and has other qualities'. But now the existence of wildly delusive perceptions, Dr. Broad maintains, lends further support to his thesis that in no case does a perceptual situation contain as a constituent the physical object which corresponds to its epistemological object; and hence the claim to external cognitive contact with such an object may very well be wrong in all perceptual situations.

In Part I of this chapter I shall consider Dr. Broad's general remarks about the 'external reference' of perceptual situations. In Part II I shall consider the relevance of the existence of delusive perception.

I. THE 'EXTERNAL REFERENCE'

I

The general remarks which Dr. Broad makes about the 'external reference' of perceptual situations may be divided into two kinds: arguments to show that we *do not*, as a matter of fact, '*infer* from the nature of the objective constituent or from any other knowledge that we may have that it is part of a larger spatio-temporal whole of a certain specific kind'; and arguments to the effect that 'it would be false as a matter of logic to maintain that this belief, in the precise form and in the actual strength in which it is held, could be justified by any known process of reasoning from any available premises'.

Now I think that Dr. Broad is perfectly correct when he says that it would be false psychologically to say that we *infer* the existence of relevant external physical objects from what is revealed to us in perception. To speak of 'unconscious inferences', he points out, means at most that we in fact reach without inference the kind of conclusion which could be defended by inference if it were challenged—though, as we have seen, Dr. Broad would deny that we actually could do this. In fact, Dr. Broad maintains:

We express the position far too intellectually, when we say that in a perceptual situation we are acquainted with an objective constituent which sensuously manifests certain qualities, and that this acquaintance gives rise to and is accompanied by a belief that the constituent is part of a larger spatio-temporal whole of a specific kind. We must remember that ignorant men, and presumably animals, perceive as well as philosophers; and we must beware of mixing up our *analysis* of the perceptual situation with the situation as it actually exists. It would be nearer the truth to say that, at the purely perceptual level, people do not have the special experience called 'belief' or 'judgment'. To believe so and so at this level really means to act as it would be reasonable to act *if* one believed so and so, and to be surprised if the action turns out to be a failure.[1]

It must be borne in mind, however, that our reasons for agreeing with Dr. Broad's contention here are somewhat different from those he holds. For we did not grant his argument in the preceding chapter that there is any reason to suppose that what we see in perceptual situations is not literally and bodily physical objects, or at least literally and bodily parts of the surface of physical objects. Dr. Broad, of course, conceives of perception as a process of going from the 'objective constituent' considered as a kind of spatially extended, two-dimensional image, having qualities only in a single modality, to the larger spatio-temporal whole of a certain specific kind, the physical object, which the situation is taken to reveal. If such were the case, there would, to be sure, be a knotty problem to unravel. But in either case, I think we may safely agree with him that it is a matter of psychological observation that the process of perception does not involve the mental phenomenon of inference.

2

I want next to consider Dr. Broad's assertion that the belief about the external reference of a perceptual situation is not only not in fact reached by inference, but could not, in the precise form and in the actual strength in which it is held, be justified by any known process of reasoning from any available premises. Dr. Broad states that he can see no way of validly inferring from the mere presence of an objective constituent, which sensuously manifests such and such qualities, that this constituent is part of a larger spatio-temporal whole which is not a constituent of

[1] *Idem*, pp. 152 f.

the situation and has other qualities. As for the argument that while this cannot be inferred with certainty from any one or from any number of perceptual situations taken separately, it might be inferred with probability from a number of such situations 'taken together and considered in their mutual relations', it is evident, Dr. Broad maintains, that even if the general validity of such inferences be admitted, they would yield a conclusion much less definite than the belief that the objective constituent of a perceptual situation is a spatio-temporal part of a larger whole which corresponds accurately to the epistemological object of the situation.

Strictly speaking, the most that could be directly inferred from a study of perceptual situations and their mutual relations is that probably such and such a perceptual situation will be accompanied by such and such others, belonging to different observers; or that it will probably be succeeded by such and such other perceptual situations, provided I make such and such movements. The notion of persistent physical objects is logically merely a hypothesis to explain such correlations between perceptual situations; and the common-sense belief that the objective constituents of perceptual situations are literally spatio-temporal parts of persistent physical objects is logically one very special form of this hypothesis. It is tolerably obvious that the actual strength of our conviction that in perception we are in direct cognitive contact with literal spatio-temporal parts of a physical object, which corresponds to the epistemological object of the situation, could not be justified by inference.[1]

Now if we were to accept Dr. Broad's conception of the objective constituent of perceptual situations as a kind of spatio-temporally extended *particular*, having qualities in a single modality, like a visual image, then I think he would be right in arguing that there is no way of validly inferring from such a particular or from a number of such particulars to the existence of the kind of things we mean by 'physical objects'. Ordinarily, we distinguish between *mere* sensory images, like after-images, hallucinatory images, and the like, and physical objects. A physical object is not merely a series or group of sensory images. With respect to any inference from P to Q, where the relation of P to Q is not one of necessary entailment, it is clear that in order to know that Q is the case, on the basis of knowing that

<hr>

[1] *Idem*, p. 152.

P is the case, it is first essential to know that P *is* somehow connected with Q. But this requires that we have independent knowledge of Q, and of the fact that P is connected with Q. One infers from hearing a certain sound, a whistle, that the afternoon train is arriving in town. But in order to do this, one must first know that there are such things as trains, and that they signal their arrival by emitting whistle blasts. Of course, other things make such sounds too, and hence there is always the possibility that the whistle one is hearing is not that of a train, but of some other of the things which make such sounds. But at any rate, if we did not know that trains existed and did make such sounds, it is clear that we could not make even a probable inference about the existence of a train, when we heard the sound of a particular whistle.

This, then, is the situation which Dr. Broad supposes we are in with respect to all perception. If all that we ever really perceive are the kinds of particulars he suggests, and we never experience physical objects as such, how can we possibly infer from the existence of these particulars the existence of physical objects? In order to do so, we should have to know independently that physical objects did exist, and that the particulars we do perceive were materially related to them. But this is precisely what we are trying to prove.

There is a certain persuasiveness about Dr. Broad's argument that is very puzzling. Even if we do not grant his conception of the objective constituent of perceptual situations as a kind of *thing* which is not to be identified literally with even a part of the surface of physical objects, there does seem to be some truth to what he is saying. We do experience at a given time and from a given position only *some* of the qualities of a part of the surface of a physical object. And we never experience all of the qualities of every bit of a physical object simultaneously. We learn what a particular object is like by seeing first one part of its surface, then another, then perhaps the various interior parts; and we feel it, touching various parts in turn; and so forth and so on. We come to know about it through having a succession of sensory experiences of the various characteristics of its parts. The same would hold true of our knowledge of *any* material object; and hence our general concept of a physical object must somehow be a product of the association of such particular perceptual

experiences occurring in fairly regular and more or less successfully predictable succession. All of this seems inescapable; and yet
Dr. Broad's conclusion seems somehow unsatisfying. For while
it may be true that the actual strength of our conviction, that in
perception we are in direct cognitive contact with literal spatio-
temporal parts of a physical object, could not be justified by
inference from objective constituents, it is also true that the
notion that persistent physical objects is logically merely a hypothesis to explain the correlations between perceptual situations,
fails to satisfy us. It seems to reduce our acquaintance with
physical objects to the level of our indirect 'knowledge by
description' of the hypothetical entities of the theoretical sciences:
the molecules of chemistry, and the atoms, electrons, etc., of
physics. All that the chemist or physicist 'really' knows is that if
we take such and such observable material substances and combine them or treat them in such and such a way, it is possible to
produce such and such observable results, which square with
and are predictable from such and such mathematical measure-
ments and calculations. Molecules, atoms, electrons, and the like
have a merely hypothetical status; they are hypotheses to account
for or explain such observations and their peculiar interrelationship.

It is obviously this type of relationship that Dr. Broad has in
mind when he says that logically the notion of persistent physical
objects is merely an hypothesis to explain the correlations between
our perceptual experiences. All we ever 'really' know by acquaintance are the succession of correlated objective constituents of
which we are sensuously aware in perceptual experience. We
experience only the effects of the kind of things we imagine
physical objects to be, and hence we can only hypothesize the
existence of physical objects as the cause or explanatory ground.
The question I want to raise, then, is whether Dr. Broad is justified in treating the relationship between perception and physical
objects, as a whole, as though it were like the relationship between
the scientist's observations and the hypothetical causes he infers.
Is Dr. Broad's 'hypothesis' really like the scientist's hypothesis?

3

In order to answer this question, it will be necessary first to
examine briefly the nature of scientific hypothesis. Now scientific

hypotheses are of many kinds. Most of them, however, permit of classification under the following three general types. (*a*) First, there are those which account for a given observable phenomenon or set of phenomena by exhibiting a causal relationship between it and another *observable* physical object or event. Thus, a given sound may be attributed to an exhaust of steam from a locomotive; a shattered window glass may be explained as the effect of a brick striking and penetrating it; and so forth. What is given as the cause of the observable condition to be explained, in hypotheses of this type, is some other observable object or event.

Now usually this other object or event which is hypothesized as the cause of the phenomenon to be explained is one which is not only observable, but is actually *familiar* to us through direct and independent experience. It is an object or event of a familiar observable kind. But frequently it happens that no known (i.e., already observed) species of object or behaviour of objects will account for the given phenomena to be explained. (*b*) This brings us to the second type of hypothesis which I want to distinguish. In such cases, the existence of a special kind of object, a kind as yet *undiscovered*, with such and such characteristics, is hypothesized. The existence and characteristics of this hypothesized entity are not known independently, as in the first type. It is merely an imagined entity having characteristics such as would account for the given phenomena to be explained. Such an hypothesized entity may be called a 'construct'. It is a *construct* because its existence and characteristics are not known independently, through direct observation, at the time of its prediction. It is an hypothetical entity whose characteristics are constructed *ad hoc* in such a way as to provide an explanation for a given problem.

As one example of this type of explanation I might suggest the gene theory in genetics. The existence of genes as carriers of hereditary predispositions was postulated to explain the mechanism of the observable facts of biological inheritance. Suppose now these hypothesized entities were actually seen with the aid of powerful microscopes. Thus, what was originally an hypothesized construct, becomes, so to speak, an actuality. The term 'gene' no longer refers to a merely hypothetical entity, but to a kind of 'thing' which we now know to 'exist'. The famous discovery of the planet Neptune by the German astronomer Galle, in 1846, as a result of the prediction based on the computations of the French astronomer Leverrier, might properly be classed as another of this type of hypothetical explanation; as may also the discovery of certain of the chemical elements predicted by Mendeléef's periodic table.

Now in the preceding examples, we were concerned with hypothetical entities of a single kind: namely, entities capable of independent and direct observation. Genes, the planet Neptune, and the predicted chemical elements are all tangible things, whose existence and characteristics were predicted from observation of relatively indirect effects. Frequently, however, scientific explanations involve as explanatory constructs hypothetical entities which are forever inaccessible to anything which even approximates direct observation. (c) This brings us to the third type of hypothesis which I want to distinguish here. The concepts of molecules, atoms, and electrons are examples of this type of explanation. These concepts are constructions which will forever remain such. At least, in the case of atoms and electrons, it seems safe to say that there will never be such a thing as 'seeing an atom' or 'seeing an electron'.

I want to elaborate upon the distinction between hypotheses of the second type and those of the third. Both involve *ad hoc* constructs whose characteristics are just those which would account for the phenomena they are invented to explain. We do not have antecedent and independent information about their existence or their characteristics. We proceed from already observable facts—the 'effects' whose explanation constitutes our problem—to the hypothesization of a certain unique 'entity', the existence of which would solve our problem. Now in explanation of the second type, the process is one of inferring the characteristics which the hypothetical entity or event must have, from the nature of its effects, and subsequently searching for and actually discovering an entity which is capable of being directly and independently observed. In hypotheses of the third type, however, this last step has not occurred. The reason for this, however, is not always the same. Sometimes the failure may be purely a practical one. Repeated search simply has failed to uncover the sought-for entity. Obviously, such failure is not always conclusive evidence of the falsity of the hypothesis that such an entity exists. While the negative results of the celebrated Michelson-Morley experiment, conducted under exacting conditions, resulted in an almost universal abandonment of the ether hypothesis, no such critical experiment seems to be possible in the case of the virus theory to explain the mechanism of that common malady known as the cold. The communicability of the cold and its course in the human system suggest a similarity to other bacterial diseases. Repeated failures to isolate the specific bacteria involved, however, have led not to the abandonment of the germ theory as an hypothesis, but to an *ad hoc* modification. It is now a *filterable* virus that is postulated. This, of course, is only a rendering of the fact that repeated search, involving filtration of the most exacting refinement known to the research worker, has (thus far) failed to reveal the hypothesized germ. In such a case the scientific enterprise proceeds thus. While some researchers continue to press the search, in the hope that some variation of conditions or the perfection of more adequate techniques and instruments will ultimately lead to the discovery, others eventually cast about for different hypothetical explanations, and the search begins anew, in different directions. It is clear in such cases that the distinction between an explanation of the second type and one of the third type may very well be only a temporal one. So long as the possibility of direct observability remains, it is always possible that what was originally merely an *ad hoc* construct will be found to be an *actual* physical object or event. Thus, the concept of the gene in genetics, as of this date merely an hypothetical construct, would pass over into the realm of the 'actual' if it came to be directly and independently observed.

While the possibility that an hypothetical construct may eventually be discovered to represent a perceptible thing or event can never logically be ruled out, often, however, there are good empirical reasons for supposing a particular construct to stand for something which could never be revealed directly and independently to perception. The concepts of molecules, atoms, and electrons in physics and chemistry do seem to be forever destined to remain on the level of mere hypothetical constructs. From the nature of the sense organs, and the psychological and physiological process of perception, it would seem that there could be no such thing as 'seeing an atom', for example. In order to be visible, an object must be capable of reflecting light in such a way that it can impinge upon the retina of the eye. By definition, an atom, or at least an electron, would not be capable of producing such an effect. Nor, by definition, could it be touched, tasted, or smelled. Although there is a temptation to suppose that these concepts stand for actual *things*, or objects, a moment's consideration will show that what they are supposed to stand for lacks, by definition, those characteristics in virtue of which any subject of discourse could be called a 'physical object'. But if the concepts do not stand for *things*, what do they stand for? For the physicist, they do not need to stand for a *thing*. They are perfectly serviceable because they function in what might be called a *metaphorical* way.

The physicist manipulates gross, microscopic objects, and derives certain observable results. In order to explain those results, which are not encompassed in the established system of explanatory concepts of mechanics or the other macroscopic branches of physics, he falls back on a kind of analogy or metaphor. His explanations might well be prefaced by the phrase, 'It is *as if*'—e.g., 'It is *as if* this piece of matter were composed of infinitely small particles (atoms)', and 'It is *as if* those hypothetical infinitely small particles (atoms) were in turn composed of still smaller particles of various kinds (electrons, protons, neutrons, mesons, etc.), revolving about in a kind of planetary system.' This kind of analogy or metaphor helps to make the puzzling clear. It yields a pictorial model based on what is familiar. It enables the physicist to 'conceive', as we say, the kind of relations he is dealing with; and in this way it enables him to make predictions which can be tested. If these predictions are verified, he concludes that he has hit upon the 'right' model. But this, of course, means only that he has chosen a happy analogy—that the bits of tangible matter he works with *do* behave under such and such conditions *as though* they were composed of ultimately small particles behaving in such and such a way. It does not mean that there are actually such things as atoms and electrons, in the sense that there are tables and chairs or even microscopic particles of dust. The physicist knows that these particles he talks about are not merely 'infinitely small' particles in the sense in which one might produce infinitely small particles by taking a very thin and sharp knife and cutting a sliver of wood first in half, then in half again, then again, and so forth and so on. For no matter how long one kept this process up, he would still not arrive at those infinitely small 'particles' which are called atoms or electrons.

THE 'EXTERNAL REFERENCE' OF PERCEPTION

To call attention to this peculiarity of hypotheses in theoretical physics is not, of course, to belittle their significance. On the contrary, it may be pointed out that physicists, working with such concepts, have accomplished so much in the way of prediction and control of the behaviour of tangible objects as to outstrip the achievements of those of their scientific brethren who work with theories and concepts having reference entirely to the directly observable. This, unfortunately, has led some non-empistemologically oriented physicists, as well as non-physicists, to venture into the dubious realm of metaphysics, in order to express their conviction that the atomic physicists are working with unquestionably 'real' objects. Logically, of course, this means only that the highly complex and neatly interrelated pattern of *observable* consequences has been so extensively and minutely verified as to make it very likely that whatever modifications of these hypothetical pictorial concepts may be necessitated by subsequent research will be of a superficial nature. The atomic physicist's conceptual notations 'work' so well as to guarantee their permanent usefulness for at least the range of phenomena they were designed to describe. Nevertheless, for our purposes, it is important to bear in mind the distinction between hypotheses of the first and second kind, and those of the third kind.

The importance of the distinction between potentially observable hypothetical entities and purely theoretical constructs may be shown by the following considerations. Let us compare the assertion that a current of water is flowing through a pipe with the assertion that a current of electricity is flowing through a wire.[1] Suppose in the first case that we are confronted with a pipe which gives certain evidences that a current of water is flowing through it. The pipe hums *as though* this were true; the indicator on the water meter, which is attached to a water wheel inside, turns *as though* a current of water was flowing within; the pipe is attached at one end to a hydrant, while from the other end a stream of water is seen to flow; when the pipe is broken in two, these phenomena cease to occur with respect to the detached portion, and are limited to the attached portion; and so forth and so on. Now suppose that in the face of this overwhelming evidence for the proposition that a current of water is actually flowing through

[1] This example is taken from J. Wisdom, 'Other Minds (III)', *Mind*, Vol. L (1941), pp. 108 f.

the pipe, the question is raised as to whether there is *actually* a current of water coursing through the pipe. From the naïve realist (scientist or layman) this question would undoubtedly evoke an exclamation of impatience, not to say of disgust and derision. But the cautious epistemologist recognizes the question as meaningful. After all, what do we *mean* by the phrase 'a current of water flowing through a pipe'? Of course, we would certainly be disinclined to say that a current of water was flowing through a pipe if all these associated phenomena were *not* observed; but it doesn't logically follow that if these phenomena are observed, a current of water is unquestionably flowing through the pipe.

Now it is clear that the epistemologist has a logical point here. The phenomena cited do not logically necessitate that 'a current of water is flowing through the pipe'. They lend a certain *probability* to the proposition, but this does not quite measure up to the certainty we do sometimes have about such matters. What is lacking is obviously a direct observation of the water flowing through the pipe. We would have to illuminate the length of pipe and peer through the open end, or perhaps to replace a section of its entire length with transparent glass. Then we could *see* the water flowing through the pipe. This would be *direct* evidence of what the proposition asserts, as opposed to *indirect* evidence—the associated phenomena. It would be meeting the defining condition of the proposition, and hence no further question could be legitimately raised. On the other hand, it is conceivable that one might cut open an opaque pipe which exhibited all the *indirect* evidence (the associated phenomena) for the presence of a water current, and find, *mirabile dictum*, that there was no water flowing through the pipe after all. This would, of course, raise the problem of what was causing the pipe to hum and the wheel to turn, etc.; but these phenomena would then have to be explained in other ways. The fact would remain that there was not a current of water flowing through the pipe. Thus, because we can specify the sort of situation meant by the assertion that despite the indirect evidence of the hum, the turning wheel, and the like, there is no water in the pipe—i.e., cutting it open and seeing that the pipe is dry—it is a *significant* doubt that is raised.

Let us consider now a similar question about a current of electricity flowing through a wire. The wire manifests all the familiar phenomena of being, as we say, 'electrified'. We touch it and experience what we call an electric shock; we attach it to an electric lamp, and the bulb lights; to a motor, and the armature revolves; the wire grows hot; the various meters all give positive readings; when we cut the wire in two, the detached half no longer exhibits these phenomena, while the portion still attached continues to do so; and so forth and so on. Suppose now that the question is raised as to whether a current of electricity is *actually* flowing through the wire that exhibits all these phenomena.

Here the logical difference between the water-pipe situation and the electric-wire situation manifests itself. What is it, we may ask, that is being doubted when the question is raised as to whether a wire which exhibits all the appropriate phenomena is *actually* electrified? Does the kind of evidence which we have in the case of the electric wire stand to the proposition that a current of electricity is passing through the wire, in the same relation as the evidence in the case of the water pipe stands to the proposition that a water current is passing through the pipe? In the latter case we were able to distinguish between indirect evidence and direct evidence—between hearing the pipe hum, seeing the meter turn, etc., and actually seeing a current of water. But obviously the distinction between indirect and direct evidence cannot be made in the same fashion with respect to the electric wire. No one expects to be able to cut open the wire and see something moving. No relevant condition or behaviour of the wire can be specified that isn't met by the wire.[1] Then is there any question as to whether or not 'an electric current is flowing through the wire'? If objections of this sort are not about terminology, what are they about? Perhaps one could object to the appropriateness of the metaphor involved in describing the phenomena associated with the wire in the terms associated with the water pipe; though the proponents of this terminology could bring to bear the behavioural similarities in justification. But at any rate, it is clear that when all the relevant kinds of phenomena are observed, the

---

[1] The objection may be raised that by a 'current of electricity' is meant a 'flow of electrons' through the wire. But this only raises the same problem on another level of theory. Translated into empirical language, this means simply that certain other 'indirect' observations associated with electron theory are supposed to be connected with the wire which exhibits these superficial phenomena. The same question that confronts us here could still be raised: when all the expected 'indirect' evidences associated with a 'flow of electrons' are verified, can we be sure that there *really* is a 'flow of electrons'?

question whether there is *really* a current of electricity flowing through the wire is lacking in sense. For it must be remembered that the conceptual language 'current of electricity' does not have an independent application, as does the phrase 'current of water'. Apart from the phenomena it was coined to denote, the phrase 'current of electricity' has no application. Here there is no distinction between direct and indirect evidence. In a given instance, one may predict, from the observation of an incomplete set of the defining characteristics of the situation 'current of electricity flowing through a wire', that further tests would reveal the remaining characteristics. But the relation between the original observation and the subsequent observation is not that of effect to observed cause—as is the relation between the associated phenomena and the independently perceptible water flowing through the pipe—but is rather that of one group of manifest behaviour to another group, which together comprise a syndrome of habitually associated phenomena. It is this syndrome that is *meant* by the assertion that a wire is carrying an electric current. The choice of the term 'electric current' was occasioned by, and serves as a reminder of, certain abstract similarities between the behaviour of pipes bearing a current of water and the behaviour of copper wires when they are attached in the proper way to a battery composed of such and such materials arranged in such and such a fashion.

4

Having outlined some of the kinds of scientific explanatory hypotheses, I want to return to Dr. Broad's treatment of the perception of physical objects in general. The question we are considering is whether or not Dr. Broad is justified in maintaining that the notion of persistent physical objects is merely an hypothesis to explain the correlations between our perceptual experiences.

Now at first glance it might seem that we had here an example of the first or second of the three types of explanatory hypotheses which we were considering. The notion of a physical object is, of course, a familiar one; and it would seem to be merely a question of whether or not our sensations were really caused by such things. It must be borne in mind, however, that Dr. Broad is not raising the question of whether or not a *particular* set of

sensations in a given situation is caused by a physical object—
i.e., whether or not a particular experience is hallucinatory. If
this were the question, it would be an empirical one, and could
be settled by further and more careful observation by the individual himself, and by the testimony of other observers. Rather,
Dr. Broad is raising the question about *all* perception. He means
to deny that we *ever* could have direct perception of physical
objects. This rules out the possibility that the concept of physical
objects is an explanatory hypothesis of even the second of our
three types; for in that type of hypothesis the explanatory construct may eventually be discovered to be an independently
perceptible object.

The position at which we have arrived seems to have been
achieved by a series of inescapable steps from Dr. Broad's
Berkeleian premises. It would seem that there aren't *really* such
things as physical objects, or, at least, that for us they are destined
forever to be at best hypothetical constructs. Apparently we are
confronted with an explanatory hypothesis of the third kind.
For there is no distinction here between direct and indirect
evidence. Granted the typical syndrome of perceptual situations,
there is no sense in the further question: Still, are there *really*
physical objects? As in the case of the electric current, there is
nothing further that we expect. Thus the concept of a physical
object seems to be merely a logical hypothesis, a construct, to
explain the correlations and mutual interrelations between perceptual situations. As Dr. Broad puts it, it is 'a Category, . . .
defined by Postulates'.[1]

There is something wrong, however, with treating the relation
of perception to physical objects as though it were that of evidence
to hypothesis, or even of phenomena to the hypothetical construct
which unites them. I want to try to show this by asking, to begin
with, what it is that we have in mind when we say that the hypothetical entities of the physicist, for example, are *only* constructs.
What do we mean when we say something is *only* an hypothesis?
What we intend by this, I submit, is to distinguish our knowledge
in a particular case from a more ideal state of knowledge which
we are capable of achieving. We distinguish the hypothetical *ad
hoc* constructs of the physicist on honorific grounds from those
directly perceivable things we call physical objects. The entities

---

[1] *The Mind and Its Place in Nature*, p. 220.

of the theoretical physicist are 'merely hypothetical' only by comparison with those things which are 'real' physical objects. If there were nothing with which to compare them, no other type of knowledge possible, it would be pointless to speak of '*hypothetical* constructs'. We would not be able to say, 'It is *as though* there were physical objects behaving in such and such a way', as the physicist does when he hypothesizes atoms and the like, or as we do when we infer the presence of a steam locomotive from hearing a certain sound. The hypothesis of the presence of a steam locomotive would not *explain* the particular sound we were hearing unless we knew that there were such things that made such sounds.

We may ask, then, when Dr. Broad states that physical objects are 'merely logical hypotheses to explain the correlations and mutual interrelations between perceptual situations': from what does he mean to differentiate them? He cannot mean to differentiate them from '*real* physical objects', obviously, for on his own argument there are not supposed to be such things—or, at least, we don't know that there are. There are only correlations of perceptual situations; and we cannot contrast a thing with itself. In that case, however, there is no sense in speaking of physical objects as 'merely hypotheses'. It is not a case of '*as if* there were physical objects'; for unless we could have some acquaintance with physical objects, we could not know the nature of the comparison that was being made.

To press this objection further, we may inquire as to just what Dr. Broad could mean by '*explaining* the correlations and mutual interrelations between perceptual situations'. When we offer an hypothesis to account for a given set of phenomena, whether the hypothesis involves a tangible object or is merely a theoretical construct, what we do is suggest that the given set of phenomena which constitute our problem may be understood by comparison or analogy with something with which we are already familiar. The phenomena with which we are confronted are reminiscent of certain other phenomena, known to be caused by the behaviour of such and such objects with which we are familiar. By analogy, we infer that the problem phenomena are caused by the behaviour of similar objects. Thus, certain phenomena associated with the concept of the atom bear a resemblance to the planetary relations in the solar system. In consequence, the physicist suggests that atomic phenomena may be understood *as though* the atom were a miniature solar system. The common cold behaves in the human organism in many ways similar to those diseases known to be caused by microscopic germs. Consequently, bacteriologists postulate the 'cold germ'.

But now, if all that we ever know or could know are 'sequences of sensations', how could there be an explanatory hypothesis that involved more than a sequence of sensations? The only kind of 'explanation' that we could understand would be one which showed how one sequence of sensations was predictably similar to another. These would be the only terms and concepts in our descriptive and explanatory language. We could not *think* any other kind of explanation. To ask for an 'explanation' of the sensation sequence that is 'outside' the sensation universe would be as nonsensical as it would be, on the common-sense position, to ask for an 'explanation' of the behavioural sequence of physical objects with the requirement that the explanation should lie 'outside' the physical universe!

The point, then, is this. Dr. Broad is mistaken in taking the relationship between perceptual situations *as a whole*, and the concept of physical objects *as a whole*, as that of evidence to hypothesis. On the common-sense view, a given series of perceptual situations may be considered as evidence for the existence of a particular object or set of objects. But this requires that the notion of physical object in general be already familiar. Otherwise we should not understand what the hypothesis was proposing. The purpose of an hypothesis is to make clear, to explain what is puzzling. This can be accomplished ultimately only through what is familiar in experience. The very demand for an explanation of a given phenomenon is a request for explication in terms of the familiar elements and processes of experience. The notion of a physical object, then, could not *explain* the correlations and interrelations between perceptual situations unless we were already somehow acquainted with physical objects in experience. In fact, it could not even be *thought*.[1] If the ultimate elements in experience were simply perceptual situations, variously correlated and interrelated, explanation would consist simply of showing

---

[1] This, of course, refers only to the concept of physical object *in general*, on the view that we *never* experience physical objects. Within the common-sense framework, we obviously can and do imagine *particular* physical objects and situations which we have never experienced.

99

how one syndrome of perceptions was correlated and interrelated like another. There would be no need for an 'explanation' of the whole perceptual series. We would neither feel the need, nor would such an 'explanation' have any meaning.

To be sure, what I am saying does not sound in the least convincing. We do feel that there would be a great deal of sense in such an explanation. I am convinced, however, that the reason we do feel this is that we are considering the matter from our present, common-sense position, in which there *is* something more ultimate and equally familiar: namely, physical objects, which causally give rise to our perceptions. This is the danger in Dr. Broad's procedure. His arguments give clear testimony to the fact that he has locked himself in the inescapable solipsist predicament *from without*. He illicitly borrows the concepts and evaluations of common sense to effect his predicament; and this is what makes his remarks so exciting. What he says is important (i.e., has *significance*) only from a common-sense position. To say that a particular entity is *merely hypothetical* tells us something only if there are other entities which are not 'merely hypothetical', with which the former may be contrasted. On the common-sense way of speaking, what the 'merely hypothetical' entities are contrasted with are *real*, tangible physical objects. On Dr. Broad's Berkeleian view, however, this standard of contrast is lacking from the start. Hence, in trying to *belittle* our knowledge of physical objects, he is really trying to have his cake and eat it.

What Dr. Broad wants to say about physical objects cannot logically be said if what he maintains is correct.[1] If he were consistently phenomenological, there would be nothing to say. Everything would be as it was—or is. There would still be those perceptions which are *merely hallucinatory*; and there would be those perceptions which we call 'perceptions of physical objects'. These are distinctions which Dr. Broad cannot very well deny. But then it is just these very distinctions which our language about perception and matter was devised to denote. That is why a sophisticated champion of common sense like Professor G. E.

---

[1] Cf. L. Wittgenstein (*Tractatus Logico-Philosophicus*):

'5.62 . . . What solipsism means, is quite correct, only it cannot be *said*, but it shows itself.'

'5.64 . . . Solipsism strictly carried out coincides with pure realism. The I in solipsism shrinks to an extensionless point and there remains the reality co-ordinated with it.'

Moore insists so tenaciously, and with justifiable righteous indignation: '*Of course* there are physical objects! What in the world can you *mean* by a "physical object" which would make it correct to say "There are no such things", or "We cannot know that there are such things"'? Professor Moore simply refuses to play the nonsensical metaphysical game of using familiar fundamental terms and phrases in radically new and different senses. For he knows that doing this only lays a verbal trap in which the metaphysician himself will unwittingly be caught. The metaphysician will want to make evaluations and draw conclusions from his special usage, which belong properly only to the original usage. This is what Dr. Broad does when he says that physical objects are logically *merely* hypotheses to explain the correlations and mutual interrelations between perceptual situations.

5

There are, of course, situations in which particular perceptual experiences may be taken as evidence for the hypothesis that a given physical object exists in a particular place. Suppose one enters a dark room and has the visual experience of a momentary patch of light. He knows, of course, that he has had such an experience, but he is not sure that there actually was a flash of light in the room. He may take his visual experience as evidence for the hypothesis that there had actually been such a light; and conversely, the hypothesis that there had been such a light may be regarded as a possible explanation to account for his perceptual experience. Suppose then that the individual proceeds to examine the room with a view to verifying his hypothesis, and discovers a lamp with faulty wiring. He suspects that this may have caused the lamp to light momentarily because of the vibrations set up by his footsteps when he entered the room. He jars it again and discovers that this produces the same kind of light flash that he saw upon entering the room. He concludes that his hypothesis of a physical source of light is correct. Though his original observation of the light flash upon entering the room was insufficient evidence on which to infer the presence of a physical source of light (because of his familiarity with after-images and other types of hallucinatory perception), when he actually sees the lamp, his hypothesis is confirmed. The presence of the lamp is for him no longer an hypothesis, but rather a fact. The very *meaning* of his hypothesis is realized when he perceives the lamp. There is nothing more that can be done; nor is there anything more that he need do.

It is just at this point, however, that Dr. Broad's 'hypothesis' is supposed to be formulated. And this is what is so puzzling about Dr. Broad's position. What is the hypothesis that remains to be verified? It is clear that when the individual had the visual experience of a flash of light upon entering the room, he was confronted with a real problem. The question was whether he had merely had an after-image, or was seeing an actual physical light. Both were real possibilities. He was claiming that the light he saw was actually a light in the room that had a physical source. Search revealed the lamp with faulty wiring. If he had not found such an object after a thorough search, he would have been justified in concluding that his visual experience was probably merely an after-image. But what is the problem when he actually finds the lamp?

Dr. Broad wants to say that the situation called 'seeing a lamp' amounts merely to having a visual experience. What we see when we 'see a lamp' is merely and at most a small spatio-temporal fragment which sensuously manifests a small selection of (visual) qualities. Further attempts at visual inspection yield only more of the same type of perceptual experiences. Thus, one can at best have only a succession of perceptual experiences, the objective constituents of which cannot properly be called a lamp. This would be true, moreover, regardless of the modality of sense in which these experiences occurred. The belief that the whole of this set of mutually correlated and interrelated perceptual experiences reveals one persistent physical object is only an hypothesis.

Now Dr. Broad's way of putting the matter suggests the following situation. Suppose that one sees an object covered in an unrevealing fashion by a large cloth. A small portion of the cloth is lifted to reveal a flat, horizontal expanse of wood, covered with a blotter. Then this portion is recovered, and another part of the cloth is lifted. This time a drawer is revealed; next a leg; and so forth and so on. The question is, what is the nature of the object beneath the cloth which is yielding all these perceptions? Is it a desk? a sewing-machine table? or what? Is it all one object, or are there several objects which are being seen in this piecemeal way?

In this case, one could offer the hypothesis that what one has been seeing is a single desk. That would account for there being a blotter, and for the object's having all the characteristics that have been observed: flat surface, drawer, legs of such and such a kind, etc. The partial glimpses that one has had would be evidence for this hypothesis. But there would still be doubt. Notice the drawer: it looks like a desk drawer. Still, sewing-machine tables often have such drawers; and so forth. The hypothesis is yet to be confirmed.

This seems to be the sort of thing that Dr. Broad conceives the perception of physical objects to be. We see only portions of objects at any given time from any given position; and we perceive them usually only by a single sense, so that we don't simultaneously perceive their other aspects and qualities. But are the cases really comparable? When, in the case of the covered object just described, we lift the cover cloth and see that it is a desk after all, obviously there is no longer any need to hypothesize. Yet Dr. Broad is still not satisfied. So long as we are perceiving the object through our senses, he wants to say that we are merely having successions of perceptual experiences. Now it is of course true that in inspecting an object we *are* 'having a succession of perceptual experiences'. But what is the relevance of the word 'merely'? What is the *more ideal* sort of knowledge he requires in order for us to be able to say that there is actually an object and that we are seeing it? It would seem that Dr. Broad wants us to perceive objects without having perceptual experiences! If we omit the word 'merely', on the other hand, his statement is a truism. It is true that seeing an object consists of having a succession of visual experiences. But this does not mean that we are merely having a series of visual experiences *instead* of seeing a physical object, as though there were merely a series of cinema images passing before our eyes. If this were the case in a particular situation, we ourselves, or other people, should soon discover the hallucinatory nature of our experience. To say that this is *always* the case, however, would be to use words so broadly as to leave them without significance. For the significance of words and of sentences lies in the distinctions we denote with them.

What is the case when we see an object can be expressed both in the language of 'succession of visual experiences', and in the language of 'seeing a physical object'. Regardless of which system of notation is used, the observable differences must be taken account of, between those experiences which are 'veridical' and those which are hallucinatory or 'non-veridical'. Just as in the case of the dispute between the Ptolemaic and the Copernican system of describing the celestial motions either notational system will really do, so in the present case we may translate freely between the 'succession of perceptual experiences' way of speaking and the 'perception of physical objects' way of speaking. Which system we choose to employ is a matter of neatness and convenience alone, the sole requirement being that we employ the system consistently, and take account of all observable differences in experience. The fact that Dr. Broad argues for the exclusive adoption of the one notational system clearly shows that he does not appreciate the purely verbal nature of the issue.

There is, it must be admitted, a certain value in doing what Dr. Broad does. He has shown, fairly accurately, what 'seeing a physical object' is like. In substituting the language of 'objective constituents' and 'succession of perceptual experiences', he is calling attention explicitly to two undeniable facts about perception and our knowledge of physical objects. The first is that perception of physical objects does proceed by 'taking the part for the whole.' The second is that our knowledge of physical objects is inescapably empirical. It is doubtful, of course, that there are many people—if any—who do not know both of these facts perfectly well. I don't suppose anyone actually thinks that he sees all over and inside a physical object at any given moment from one single position, or that he feels, tastes, and smells the object when he is only looking at it. Nor do I suppose anyone thinks that knowledge about physical objects is to be attained in any other way than through empirical observation. Yet it is probably well to be reminded of these facts from time to time. It helps to remind us and warn us of how we may fall into error. For it occasionally turns out that the directly perceived aspect of an object is a misleading clue to the nature of the object. But this is not at all the kind of possibility Dr. Broad is concerned with.

What are we to say, then, concerning Dr. Broad's observation that there is no way of validly inferring from the mere presence of an objective constituent which sensuously manifests such and such qualities that this is a constituent of a larger spatio-temporal whole which is not a constituent of the situation, and which has other qualities? Though, for the reasons which I have presented in some detail, I cannot agree with what Dr. Broad wants to make of this fact, I think he is perfectly correct in saying this. I fail to see, however, that this constitutes a real problem for epistemology. For perceptual knowledge is, after all empirical knowledge, and not purely a matter of logical deduction. So long as we see only a part of a physical object, we cannot infer with logical necessity the characteristics of the unseen portion, or the qualities not sensuously revealed.

This is true of all empirical matters. We cannot purely logically infer the correlation of two phenomena. There is no logical contradiction involved in saying that one phenomenon occurs but the other does not. Whether or not they are co-present in any given situation is something which can be said with certainty only after recourse to empirical observation. This does not mean, however, that our convictions about empirical correlations are wholly without ground. Our convictions in such matters are based upon careful, repeated observation, supplemented by insight into the principles of interconnection which afford more than a grossly statistical justification to our predictions of continued correlation. It is just this which we mean when we speak of *empirical evidence* for a causal generalization, for example. Similarly, through experience, we become familiar with the behaviour of physical objects. If our perceptual judgments about physical objects based on partial perceptions were not in fact dependable, we should not have developed the habits of judgment and speech which we do have. Were everyday life like a Hollywood movie set, we should soon learn to take care in our speech and judgment lest we mistake what is only an artificial façade for a substantial building. In any case, our knowledge of the physical world is ultimately empirical; and though on occasion there may be some uncertainty as to whether our perceptual experience is veridical or delusive, further observation will decide the matter.

II. THE RELEVANCE OF DELUSIVE PERCEPTION

I

Dr. Broad next turns to consider the relevance of delusive perceptual situations for the analysis of the relationship between epistemological object and ontological object. The drunkard, he points out, says that he sees pink rats, and he *means* by this the same thing, *mutatis mutandis*, as the sober man means when he says, for example, that he sees a brown penny.

. . . The former means by 'pink rats' something which lasts beyond the duration of the perceptual situation, which could be felt as well as seen, which could be seen and felt by other men, which could eat corn and excite fox-terriers, and so on. We call this perceptual situation 'delusive' because none of these expectations, which form an essential factor in the situation, are verified by the contemporary perceptions of other observers or by the subsequent perceptions of the drunkard himself. We must remember that, although no amount of perceptual verification can prove that the objective constituent of a perceptual situation *is* a part of a physical object of a certain specified kind, complete failure of such verification may make the contradictory of this almost certain. It may be doubtful whether there are such things as pennies, in the sense in which the unphilosophical teetotaller asserts that there are; and it may be doubtful whether the objective constituent of the situation which we call 'the teetotaller's perception of a penny' is literally part of a penny, as he believes it to be. But it is practically certain that there are no such things as pink rats, in the sense in which the unphilosophical drunkard asserts that there are, when he is in the situation called 'seeing pink rats'.[1]

Now Dr. Broad is certainly correct in asserting that we can determine that certain perceptual experiences are delusive, and that there are no such things as pink rats in the sense in which the drunkard suffering from hallucination says that there are. And I think it may very likely be the case that when the drunkard sincerely asserts that he is seeing pink rats, he does mean to say the same sort of thing, *mutatis mutandis*, as the sober man does when the latter asserts that he is seeing, for instance, a brown penny. I am puzzled, however, by Dr. Broad's statement that though no amount of perceptual verification can prove that the objective constituent of a perceptual situation *is* a part of a physical object of a certain specified kind, complete failure of such verification may make the contradictory of this almost certain. It is indeed true that complete failure of verification may make the contradictory 'almost certain'; but it is not at all clear that on the same type of empirical evidence equal certainty cannot be achieved with respect to the original affirmative proposition.

[1] *The Mind and Its Place in Nature*, p. 155.

The reason that Dr. Broad contents himself with the statement that the contradictory can be made '*almost* certain', I take it, is that inasmuch as this is an empirical matter, something short of *logical* necessity must be the ultimate that can be achieved in verification. But, then, isn't this also true of the affirmative proposition? Logical necessity is similarly unattainable; but cannot there be practical certainty? Why is it, we may ask, that we *can* be almost certain that the objective constituent of a perceptual situation is *not* a part of a physical object of a certain specified kind? The answer, of course, is that we know the meaning of a sentence which asserts a proposition to that effect—which is to say, we know what *would be the case*, empirically, if it was true that the objective constituent was not a part of the kind of physical object we had in mind. When we assert that the thing we are seeing, which looks like a book, is not a book, but is perhaps a bonbon container designed to look like a book from the outside, we expect when we open the cover to find it hollow and filled with candy, instead of with printed pages. We trust the 'evidence' of our senses because, in the first place, we have no reason to suppose that the situation is further delusive; and secondly, because what we mean to assert is an empirical proposition for which the testimony of the senses is the only really relevant kind of evidence. Thus, when we corroborate the testimony of our eyes by further visual inspection, and by feeling the hollow interior, and perhaps even by sampling the candy, we have all the evidence we need that what we first took to be a book is really a bonbon container.

But, now, is it not in precisely the same way that we verify, on the proper occasion, that our perceptual judgments are correct? We know what a book is, and we know what we mean by 'seeing a book'. We pick it up, open it, read its printed pages, and thereby establish that it *is* a book at which we are looking, and not something else. Our judgment has been empirically verified. In fact, in one sense, it might be argued with no little justification that under such circumstances it is *logically necessary* that the proposition be recognized as true. For it is a case of just the sort of thing originally meant, demonstrably, by 'seeing a book'.

I fail to see how the matter is different with regard to an affirmative judgment of perception from what is the case with regard to its contradictory. Consider how we determine that a given perceptual situation is delusive. We make a judgment, on the basis of what we have perceived, which entails certain further empirical consequences. When we come to examine the object further, we find that our expectations are not realized. We conclude that our original perceptual judgment was mistaken. But obviously, in order to conclude this, we must regard our second observation as veridical. In order to conclude that it is *not* a book which we are seeing, we must be satisfied that it *is* a bonbon container. To put the matter another way, we may ask how it is that we can determine that a given perceptual situation is delusive save by knowing what *would* be the case if it were not delusive, and seeing that not this but something else is the case? But from whence comes our expectation as to what *should* be the case if our perceptual judgment is to be correct? This question is especially pertinent when the issue is not whether what we are seeing is this object rather than that, but rather whether we *ever* see physical objects. The question is pertinent enough when we ask how it is that we know what to expect in terms of empirical consequences when we judge that we are seeing a book. Obviously we should not know what to expect unless we had previously had some acquaintance with books, and knew what 'seeing a book' is like. It sometimes happens, however, that our expectations are based on our 'knowledge by description' of what certain objects which we have never personally seen are like. But this 'knowledge by description' is, of course, ultimately derived from *someone's* 'knowledge by acquaintance'. In any event, however, when the issue is whether *any* perception ever reveals a physical object, if we had not *some*times perceived a physical object, it is clear that we could not know that a given experience was not a perception of an actual physical object. If the matter is not to be wholly a verbal one, there must be some empirical basis for the criteria we employ in deciding that a given perceptual experience is not a perception of a physical object. Otherwise, we should have no reason to expect physical objects to yield 'veridical' patterns of perceptions rather than 'delusive' patterns. Inasmuch as we should know nothing about the nature of physical objects, we should just as soon expect physical objects to behave like the objects of hallucinatory experience, disappearing and reappearing and changing in appearance without rhyme or reason. In that case, however, what happens to the distinction between 'veridical' perception and 'hallucination'? With that distinction obliterated, Dr. Broad's 'argument from delusive perception' dissipates into thin air.

2

Let us consider now just what importance Dr. Broad attaches for his analysis to the existence of delusive perceptual situations of the pink-rat kind.

(*a*) For one thing, says Dr. Broad, it supports the observation, made somewhat above, that language is a partly misleading guide to the analysis of perceptual situations.

The drunkard says 'I see a pink rat', just as the sober man says 'I see a brown penny'; and, *mutatis mutandis*, they mean exactly the same kind of thing by their two statements. So long as we follow the suggestions of language, there is just as much reason for holding that a pink rat is a constituent of the drunkard's perceptual situation as for holding that a brown penny is a constituent of the sober man's perceptual situation. But this analysis *must* be wrong in the former case, since there is almost certainly no pink rat to be a constituent of anything. And, since there is no relevant internal difference between the veridical and the delusive perceptual situation, it is reasonable to suppose that in no case does a perceptual situation contain as a constituent the physical object which corresponds to its epistemological object, when when there is such a physical object.[1]

Now it should be noticed, in the first place, that the way in which 'language is a partly misleading guide to the analysis of perceptual situations', at least so far as the present argument is concerned, is quite different from what Dr. Broad would have us believe. All that follows from the fact that drunkards say 'I see a pink rat', and mean the same thing by this, *mutatis mutandis*, as the sober man does when he says 'I see a brown penny', is that language is a misleading guide to the analysis of *delusive* perceptual situations. It may very well be that language is a misleading guide to the analysis of delusive perceptual situations, while it is a perfectly accurate guide to the analysis of veridical perceptual situations; and, in fact, I want to contend just this.

The second objection which I want to raise concerns Dr. Broad's assertion that 'there is no relevant internal difference

---

[1] *Idem*, p. 156.

between the veridical and the delusive perceptual situation'. Since this is true, Dr. Broad maintains, 'it is reasonable to suppose that in no case does a perceptual situation contain as a constituent the physical object which corresponds to its epistemological object; even when there is such a physical object'. Now I do not think that this is precisely the point which Dr. Broad really intends to make here.[1] For he has already argued, from an artificially narrow definition of 'perceptual situation' and 'objective constituent', as I have shown, that a perceptual situation could not in any case 'contain as a constituent' anything more than just that part of the surface of the whole physical object which is immediately and sensuously revealed. Thus, the point which he means to make here, I believe, is rather that, since there is no such thing as a pink rat to be the constituent of the drunkard's delusive perceptual situation, and since there is no relevant internal difference between the veridical and the delusive perceptual situation, it is reasonable to suppose that in *no* case does a perceptual situation contain as a constituent *even a part of the surface of* the physical object which corresponds to its epistemological object, even when there is such an object. It should be understood that this is the point which I mean to argue, whether or not I explicitly distinguish in my language between the whole physical object and the immediately perceptible part of it.

Now it seems to me that Dr. Broad has here committed an error in reasoning that is so obvious as to give one to wonder if he really meant to say just what he does. From the fact that there are delusive perceptual situations whose epistemological objects do not correspond to any ontological object in the external world,

---

[1] In Sec. 8 of the preceding chapter, I considered the possibility that Dr. Broad means by a 'perceptual situation' only a sensory experience—what, in common-sense terms, might be denoted as the purely sensory aspect of a situation involving a physical object, say a chair, and a perceiving subject visually aware of the chair. In that case, of course, the 'perceptual situation' could not, in any case, correctly be said literally to contain the chair as a constituent; and Dr. Broad's point, albeit a merely verbal one, would certainly be correct. But then, too, his further remarks, including those I am considering here, would either be unnecessary or irrelevant. Though there is good reason, as I have indicated, to believe that this is just what Dr. Broad does mean by a 'perceptual situation', the fact that he goes on to make the point which he makes here would also seem to indicate that he means to hold this view in temporary abeyance while considering the present, independent argument. Thus, it behoves us to consider his present argument seriously, apart from this question-begging definition of the 'perceptual situation'.

and from the added fact that there is 'no relevant internal differ-ence' between delusive and veridical perceptual situations, it is obvious that all that Dr. Broad is entitled to conclude, reasonably, is that in no case can one *know* from a given perceptual situation alone whether or not it contains as a constituent the physical object which corresponds to its epistemological object. This, of course, is quite a different matter from concluding that in no case *does* a perceptual situation contain such an object as its constituent. To argue the latter proposition on these premises would be as absurd as it would be to argue that because a hen might occasionally lay an egg which did not contain a yolk, and there would be no relevant difference in superficial appearance between such eggs and those which *are* held to contain yolks, that therefore it would be reasonable to suppose that no eggs contain yolks!

Supposing, however, that Dr. Broad's argument is that we cannot *know* with respect to any given perceptual situation whether or not it contains as a constituent the physical object which corresponds to its epistemological object, to what extent can we accept this argument? To begin with, I think that Dr. Broad is probably right in holding that there is 'no relevant internal difference' between the veridical and the delusive per-ceptual situation. At least, I suppose, drunkards who suffer from hallucinations of pink rats are not able to distinguish such perceptual situations, at the moment they are the subject of them, from veridical perceptual situations. But the importance of this is not at all clear. For it isn't on the basis of single, isolated, momentary perceptual situations that the distinction between veridical and delusive perception is generally made. The point is rather that if one *continued* to 'look' at an hallucinatory 'object', attempted to verify it through his other senses and through the testimony of other human observers and physical instruments, he would soon discover that its behaviour was different from that of physical objects, and the hallucinatory nature of his experience would thus be revealed.

In this issue, of course, it is very important just how the term 'perceptual situation' is defined. Dr. Broad does not make it entirely plain whether he would term a situation in which an individual was simultaneously seeing, touching, and hearing a bell *one* perceptual situation or three separate and distinct perceptual situations. It is clear that if he considered the simultaneous elements as comprising a single perceptual situation, as they are for the individual observer, there *would* be relevant discernible differences between veridical and delusive perceptual situations. If, however, as I suspect, Dr. Broad means to define the term 'perceptual situation' in such a way as to rule out corroborating perceptions, then the point which he wins on this narrow and artificial definition is purely a verbal one. Whether or not a given perception is veridical is, of course, an empirical matter. It is something which can be determined only by further observation. In that case, Dr. Broad's argument should occasion no concern. For it is common knowledge that the way to make certain that one is actually seeing a physical object and is not the victim of a delusion is to make use of the criteria which Dr. Broad, by his arbitrary definition of the 'perceptual situation,' rules out—namely, looking some more, touching, comparing one's observations with those of others, employing physical instruments, and the like. In this way one can determine that he is having a veridical perception of a physical object—or that he is not, as the case may be.

Finally, it seems to me that if the absence of a physical object corresponding to what one thinks he is seeing in hallucinatory visual perception is good reason to conclude that the perceptual situation does not contain a physical object as a constituent, then, on the same argument, the very presence of such an object in veridical perception should entitle one to conclude that this situation *does* contain a physical object as a constituent. At least, Dr. Broad has not yet satisfactorily established this to be false, in the sense that it would ordinarily be claimed. And the very fact that he cites hallucinatory cases in support of his thesis shows that he knows the difference between delusive cases in which there is no ontological object corresponding to the epistemological object, and veridical cases in which there is.

3

(*b*) The second point which Dr. Broad wants to argue on the basis of the existence of wildly delusive perceptual situations (hallucinations) is somewhat similar to his first. This is that inasmuch as the admitted, though often unverbalized, claim to be part of a physical object is not met with respect to the objective constituents of hallucinatory perceptual situations, and inasmuch as there is no internal distinction between these cases and those in which the same kind of claim is made and met, the claim may be wrong in all. Thus, not only is the alleged external object not literally part of the objective constituent, according to Dr. Broad, but there may not even be an external object.

Each perceptual situation, says Dr. Broad, contains an objective constituent of a characteristic kind; and in each case this is bound up with the belief that this constituent is 'part of a larger and more enduring whole which possesses other qualities beside those which are sensuously manifested in the situation'. Though this practical belief, which 'goes beyond the immediate situation and its contents', is certainly wrong in the case of hallucinations, so far as we have yet seen, Dr. Broad admits, it might be right in so-called veridical perceptual situations. But, he maintains, there is absolutely nothing in the two kinds of situations *as such* to distinguish the case where the belief is certainly false from the case where it is possibly true.

Now if there had been no delusive perceptual situations, Dr. Broad argues, it might have been held that every perceptual situation is as such accompanied by an infallible revelation that its objective constituent is part of a larger and more enduring whole of a certain kind. All perceptual situations involve this claim; and if there had been no reason to suppose that the claim is ever false, why then there would be no reason to consider it as merely a claim. The fact that there are delusive perceptual situations of the pink-rat sort, however, cuts out this alternative. The claim in the case of pink rats is of precisely the same kind as and of equal strength to that made when teetotallers perceive pennies. But if it be false in *some* cases, says Dr. Broad, and there is nothing in the two situations as such to distinguish them, it cannot be accepted as true merely at its face value in *any* case. Thus, inasmuch as he has already argued that the external reference of a perceptual situation cannot be regarded as a valid logical inference from the existence of the situation and the nature of its objective constituent, Dr. Broad considers it a real possibility that the claim to external reference may be wrong in all perceptual situations.

Of course, Dr. Broad observes, if this claim be 'watered down' enough, it may be put so generally and loosely as to defy refutation:

If we claim merely that the objective constituents in all perceptual situations are correlated in *some* way with *something* larger and more enduring than themselves, and that every variation in the former is a sign of a change of *some* kind *somewhere or other* in the latter, we can hardly be refuted. There is, no doubt, some such correlation between the objective constituent of the drunkard's perceptual situation and the alcohol in his stomach or something that is happening in his brain. But I think it is perfectly clear that perceptual situations do involve a more specific claim than this; and that, since this specific claim is certainly wrong in some cases and since there is no internal distinction between these cases and others, it may be wrong in all.[1]

Here again the argument quite obviously rests on Dr. Broad's definition of the limits of a single perceptual situation. If he chooses the narrow definition as described above, and if it be granted that there are hallucinatory perceptual situations indistinguishable on their face from veridical ones, then I think we must grant that we could not say of a given perceptual situation, taken in isolation, whether or not it was veridical. There is also a sense in which Dr. Broad's suggestion that the claim to external reference 'may be wrong in *all* cases'. The sense in which this is right, however, is that in which this phrase is taken to mean 'may be wrong in *any* case'. As I have already noted, this is an empirical matter, and it is not only logically possible that a given perceptual experience should be delusive, but in fact, as Dr. Broad has himself indicated, we *know* that some are.

To argue, however, that because each momentary perceptual experience, taken by itself, *may* be fallacious, therefore the *whole* of perceptual experience is suspect, is a perfect example of the classic 'material fallacy' known as the fallacy of *composition*. It is like arguing that because each member of a trial jury is fallible, nothing is gained by the mere addition of twelve carefully selected men; or that because each individual summation of a column of figures by anyone may be in error, no advantage is gained by having several men repeat the calculation, even when they all agree. And in another respect, it is like arguing that because adding several inches to the height of any member of a group of persons lined up according to height would move that

[1] *The Mind and Its Place in Nature*, p. 157.

man nearer to the high end of the line, therefore adding the same number of inches to the heights of every member of the group would move them *all* nearer to the high end of the line.

Let us see what this comes to with respect to the specific argument at hand. To begin with the second aspect of the fallacy, it is logically nonsense, as I have argued before, to hold that *all* perceptions are delusive. For we determine that some perceptual situations are delusive only by comparing them with others which we know to be veridical This is what we *mean* by describing a perception as 'delusive'. Obviously it is a *relative* concept. Thus, to say that *all* perception is delusive is to rob the term of its very significance. It is to overlook the differences which the terms 'veridical' and 'delusive' were coined to distinguish. In doing this, it may be pointed out, Dr. Broad is somewhat in the position of the man who believed in dreams, and then dreamt that dreams are not to be trusted! For he seems to be arguing explicitly from the discernible difference between delusive and veridical perceptual situations, to the conclusion that there is no discernible difference between delusive and veridical perceptual situations. One wonders, naturally, why he does not continue to avail himself of the same methods of discernment which originally suggested to him his paradoxical conclusion.

This brings us to the first-mentioned aspect of the fallacy. Dr. Broad argues that there is nothing in the two situations *as such* to distinguish the case where the belief is certainly false from the case where it is possibly true. There is, he says, no relevant *internal* difference between the two cases. This, as I have admitted, may well be true. But now obviously we could not know that the belief is 'certainly false' in a given perceptual situation, merely from considering the momentary situation *as such*. It should not be surprising, then, that we cannot know whether or not the belief is correct, on the same grounds. After all, something *is* gained by having twelve carefully selected men on a jury instead of only one; and it *does* make a difference if several men repeat a calculation and arrive at equivalent results. Similarly, we verify our perceptions by succeeding observations, over a period of time that is long enough to detect the characteristic 'instability', etc., which hallucinatory 'objects' exhibit, and which perceptions of actual physical objects do not. We corroborate our perceptions by our other senses and by the testimony of others. And, simultaneously, we bring to bear knowledge of antecedent circumstances with respect to ourselves and our physiological and mental condition, and with respect to the external objective situation.

If all the relevant criteria by means of which we ascertain which of our perceptual experiences are veridical, and which hallucinatory, are arbitrarily ruled out, why, then, of course we have no grounds for deciding. But what is the justification for so ruling them out? Dr. Broad's answer, as we saw in Part I, Section 2, of the present chapter, is that the hypothesis of external physical objects cannot be validly inferred from any one or from any number of perceptual situations taken separately, or from a number of such situations 'taken together and considered in their mutual relations'. And hence he wants to hold that successive perceptions are not relevant to the issue at hand. I have shown, however, that the relationship between successive perceptions and physical objects cannot, in general, be correctly considered as that of evidence to hypothesis; and hence the fact that the presence of an external physical object cannot be *inferred* from perceptual situations constitutes no good reason for rejecting the latter as relevant means for distinguishing between veridical and delusive perception. I conclude, therefore, that Dr. Broad has failed to show that we can never know that a perceptual situation is veridical—that, specifically, we are actually seeing a physical object.

CHAPTER IV

THE 'LOGICAL QUESTION' AND THE ALTERNATIVE THEORIES

D R. BROAD claims to have shown thus far three things about the perception of physical objects, all inimical to common sense.[1] These are (a) that the external object as such is never a constituent of the perceptual situation; (b) that the claim that the objective constituent of a perceptual situation is in fact literally part of a larger external object of a certain specific kind, having other qualities beside those which are sensuously manifested in the situation, can never be accepted at its face-value, because it is certainly sometimes false in situations which differ in no relevant internal respect from those in which it might be true; and (c) that this claim cannot be proved to be true as it stands by logical inference from any premises which are available to us.

In reply, it will be recalled, I argued that the first claim followed only from the fact that Dr. Broad defines 'perceptual situation' and 'objective constituent' so as to include only sensory experience and exclude entirely external physical objects, or, at least, so as to exclude all but the immediately sensible qualities of that portion of the surface of an object which is sensuously revealed to the perceiver in a single sense modality at a given moment. Similarly, I showed that the second claim followed only because Dr. Broad arbitrarily rules out the criteria which we actually do employ in determining whether perceptual experiences are veridical or hallucinatory. The fact that the objective constituents of perceptual situations of the latter type cannot be identified

[1] *The Mind and Its Place in Nature*, p. 158.

117

as literally parts of physical objects, I argued, is no reason to suppose that the objective constituents of veridical perceptual situations cannot be so identified either. The fact that the claim of a single isolated perception to veridicality cannot be accepted at its face-value is no reason to suppose that we *never* know whether or not it is veridical. Finally, with respect to the third claim, the upshot of the discussion was that while the suggestion that *all* perceptual situations are non-veridical is logically non-sensical, it is not surprising that the claim to external reference which all perceptual situations make cannot be proved to be true by logical inference; for whether or not a given perception is veridical is a matter not of logical inference, but rather of *empirical* verification.

In the present chapter I want to discuss the first of two major difficulties which Dr. Broad finds in the common-sense notion of the perception of physical objects, with respect to the issue of whether or not the objective constituents of perceptual situations are ever literally identical with even parts of the surfaces of 'external' physical objects. One of these difficulties Dr. Broad terms 'logical'; the other, 'causal'. In this chapter I shall discuss two of the alternative theories of sense-perception and matter which Dr. Broad proposes as possible solutions to the difficulty he alleges: namely, the *Theory of Multiple Inherence* and the *Multiple Relation Theory of Appearing*. The following chapter will take up the 'causal' problem. In the sixth and final chapter I shall discuss the third of the three alternative theories which Dr. Broad proposes, and which he himself favours: the *Sensum Theory*.

I

The 'logical' question which Dr. Broad raises concerns the apparent inconsistency of perceptual appearances. In view of the fact that a physical object seems to differ in size, shape, and colour for simultaneous different observers, or for one and the same observer as he moves about, what is required, Dr. Broad maintains, if we are to hold on to the common-sense view that the objective constituents of perceptual situations are literally parts of external objects, is a reconsideration of the formal character-istics of the relation of these attributes to the objective constituents of perceptual situations and to physical objects.

He asks whether we can hold that the claim is *ever* true that the objective constituent of a perceptual situation is in fact 'literally a part of a certain specific kind of object, having other qualities beside those which are sensuously manifested in the situation'.[1] On the supposition that the claim is true, Dr. Broad contends that he can prove that we are tied down to two alternatives, 'neither of which accords very well with common sense'. These are that the objective constituent of a visual situation does not have some of the properties which it seems, on careful inspection, to have, and does have properties inconsistent with these; or that the larger external whole of which it is a part is so different from what it is commonly supposed to be that it hardly deserves the name of 'physical object'. I want to consider the arguments which Dr. Broad offers in support of his contention.

In presenting his proof that we are tied to these alternatives if we attempt to maintain the common-sense notion that the objective constituents of perceptual situations may be literally parts of larger external objects, Dr. Broad cites the familiar case of observing a penny. A penny, he says, is believed by common sense to be a round flat object whose size and shape are independent of the observer, his position, and his movements. A given observer may move about, and may hold that in all the perceptual situations in which he is placed he sees the whole of the top of a certain penny. If the observer carefully inspects the objective constituents of these perceptual situations, however, says Dr. Broad, he will certainly find that they seem to be of different shapes and sizes and of different colours or shades. With respect to shape, for example, most of them will seem elliptical and not round, and the direction of their major axes and their eccentricities will seem to vary as he moves. Now, says Dr. Broad, if these objective constituents are to be identified with 'different short slices of the history of the top of the penny', one of two views must be taken. (*a*) One alternative is to suppose that these objective constituents *really are* all round and all of one size, although they *seem*, on careful inspection, to be elliptical and of various sizes and eccentricities. (*b*) The other alternative is to suppose that the penny is not of constant size and shape, as is commonly believed, but that it varies as the observer walks about.[2]

Now the latter alternative, Dr. Broad remarks, might be the

[1] *Ibid.*   [2] *Idem*, pp. 158 f.

reasonable one to take if the successive visual situations of only one observer had to be considered. But the neutrality and publicity which are part of the notion of a physical object require that we take into account the reports of a number of simultaneous observers who agree that they are all seeing the whole of the top of the same penny. If one of these observers stands still, while another moves about, the result is that the objective constituent of the stationary observer's perceptual situation will seem constant in size and shape, while the objective constituents of the moving observer's successive perceptual situations will seem to differ in size and shape. Evidently, says Dr. Broad, if we suppose that these objective constituents really do have the characteristics which they seem to have—that the observers really are seeing the whole of the top of the same penny; and that the objective constituents of their respective perceptual situations really are identical with a slice of the history of the penny—we shall have to suppose that the penny *both* changes and keeps constant in shape and size during the same stretch of time. And this, says Dr. Broad, seems at first sight impossible.[1]

A similar difficulty confronts us, Dr. Broad continues, when we consider the situation in which a man feels a penny, and at the same time moves his head about while he continues to inspect the penny. While the objective constituent of the tactual situation will seem to be constant in shape and size, those of the successive visual situations will seem on inspection to differ in shape and size. Now, says Dr. Broad, common sense holds that it is the same surface which we see and which we touch; though certain non-spatial qualities, such as colour, are sensuously manifested only in one kind of situation. Thus, if we try to keep the common-sense view that the objective constituents of some visual situations are literally spatio-temporal parts of a certain physical object which we are said to be 'seeing', Dr. Broad concludes, we must hold either (*a*) that the objective constituents of some perceptual situations have certain qualities which differ from and are inconsistent with those which they seem on careful inspection to have, or (*b*) that one and the same surface can vary and keep constant in shape and size within the same stretch of time.

On the other hand, Dr. Broad suggests, there is a third alternative. (*c*) We may drop the common-sense view that the objective

---

[1] *Idem,* p. 159.

constituent of a visual situation may be, and in some cases actually is, literally a spatio-temporal part of a certain physical object which we are said to be 'seeing'.[1]

Corresponding to the three alternatives just presented, Dr. Broad proceeds to develop three theories: (a) 'The Multiple Relation Theory of Appearing', (b) 'The Theory of Multiple Inherence', and (c) 'The Sensum Theory'. In this chapter, as I have said, I shall consider, with respect to the 'logical' problem they are designed to solve, the first two theories, which allow the common-sense view that the objective constituents of some visual situations are literally spatio-temporal parts of physical objects.

2

The Theory of Multiple Inherence and the Multiple Relation Theory of Appearing are both designed to keep the common-sense view that the objective constituents of some visual situations are literally spatio-temporal parts of the particular physical object which we are said to be seeing. The Multiple Inherence Theory meets this requirement by replying to the problem of the apparent inconsistency of perceptual judgments with the postulation that the physical object can be both constant and variable in its spatial characteristics within the same stretch of time. The Multiple Relation Theory meets the problem by holding that the objective constituents of the supposedly incompatible perceptual situations can have qualities which are different from and inconsistent with those which they seem on careful inspection to have.

According to the Multiple Inherence Theory, we must distinguish between the 'sensible' and the 'physical' inherence of a quality, colour, for example, in a place. The former, Dr. Broad tells us,[2] is the fundamental and indefinable relation, on this theory; and it is irreducibly triadic, involving an essential reference to the pervading shade of colour, the pervaded region, and the region of projection—i.e., the place *from* which the pervaded region appears to be pervaded by the pervading shade of colour. 'Physical' inherence, on the other hand, is a two-term relation on this theory; but it is not ultimate, being definable in terms of the

1 *Idem*, pp. 160 f.
2 *Idem*, p. 163.

former. The full statement of this definition, Dr. Broad writes, would not, I think differ very much from the following: '*s* is physically red' means 'From every place which is physically occupied by a normal human brain and nervous system in a normal condition and is near enough to *s* some shade of red sensibly inheres in *s*.'[1]

With these definitions, Dr. Broad believes, it is then possible to maintain the common-sense view that a physical object cannot have two different colours at once. The point would be that two different colours cannot *sensibly* inhere in the same place *from the same place* at once; nor can they *physically* inhere in the same place at once; but two different colours or different shades of the same colour can *sensibly* inhere in the same place from *different* places at once. Thus, it would be entirely possible for two different individuals at different places at the same time to perceive two different colours or shades of the same colour pervading a given region.

In similar fashion, Dr. Broad tells us, the Theory of Multiple Inherence can, in his opinion, meet the more difficult yet inescapable question of simultaneous discrepant perceptual judgments of size and shape, which arise, for example, when a circular penny appears to different observers, viewing it at once from different positions, to have different shapes and sizes, etc. There is, he argues, a defensible distinction which can be made between a 'sensible form' and a 'geometrical property', corresponding to the distinction between the sensible and physical pervasion or inherence of colour in a given place. Thus, while the *geometric* shape of a region may be said to be an intrinsic property of that region, and the region could have only one *geometric* shape at any given time, it could have different *sensible* forms from different places at once. The relation of being sensibly 'informed', Dr. Broad observes, would, as with sensibly 'pervaded', in the case of colour, be irreducibly triadic. Thus, the Theory of Multiple Inherence appears to meet the 'logical' problem which it is designed to answer.

The Multiple Relation Theory of Appearing, Dr. Broad observes, bears a close formal analogy to the Theory of Multiple Inherence. The Multiple Inherence Theory supposes that colours 'inhere' triadically in places from places, and that sensible forms

[1] *Idem*, p. 165.

triadically 'inform' regions from regions; and it holds that 'physical' inherence and 'geometric' shape are reducible to the more fundamental triadic relations. Now while the Multiple Relation Theory allows that if a colour really did inhere in anything, it would inhere dyadically, as common sense supposes, Dr. Broad tells us, it has to assume a fundamental relation of 'appearing', which must be at least triadic.[1] Thus, on this theory, a distinction is made, with respect to characteristics like colour, shape, etc., between propositions of the form 'This *is* red', and those of the form 'This *looks* red from here'. This distinction, Dr. Broad tells us, is the concession which the Multiple Relation Theory must make in order to deal with the known facts. For in order to maintain the common-sense view that the objective constituents of at least some visual situations are literally spatio-temporal parts of physical objects, in the face of apparent discrepancies in perceptual judgments, it has to assume that the objective constituent of a visual situation can seem from a place to have characteristics which are other than and incompatible with the characteristics which it does have.

The top of a penny, for example, seems to have a number of different shades of the same colour (under different conditions), and may even seem to have a number of different colours, from different places occupied by different observers. Obviously, Dr. Broad observes, if the top of a penny literally has a certain colour dyadically, it can have only one shade of one colour. It follows, then, that if a penny literally and dyadically possesses any colour, the colour which it *has* must differ from all but one of the colours or shades which it *seems* to have; and it may differ from all of them.[2] The same remarks, Dr. Broad points out, apply, on this theory, to shape, size, and position.

These, then, in brief, are the two theories which will permit us to maintain the common-sense notion that the objective constituents of some visual situations are literally spatio-temporal parts of the physical objects which we suppose ourselves to be seeing. Both theories allow, Dr. Broad sums up for us, that, under suitable conditions, it may be true that there is a common objective constituent to the visual situations of a number of observers who say that they are 'seeing the same object'. Both

[1] *Idem*, p. 178.
[2] *Idem*, p. 179.

allow that there is, under suitable conditions, a common objective constituent to the visual and tactual situations of an observer who says that he is 'seeing and feeling the same object'. And both allow that, under suitable conditions, this common objective constituent may be literally a spatio-temporal part of the object which the various observers say that they are 'seeing and feeling'. At this point, however, says Dr. Broad, each theory diverges from common sense in a different direction. The Multiple Inherence Theory allows that the objective constituent really does have those characteristics which it seems on careful inspection by each observer to have. But it can allow this only by supposing that these characteristics inhere in the objective constituent triadically—that is, Dr. Broad points out, in a way never contemplated by common sense. The Multiple Relation Theory of Appearing, on the other hand, allows that *if* the objective constituent did have such characteristics as it seems to have, they *would* inhere in it in the ordinary dyadic way which common sense recognizes. But, he notes, it can allow this only by supposing that most, if not all, of the determinate characteristics which the objective constituent seems on careful inspection to have do not in fact inhere in it.[1]

3

I want now to consider whether or not the 'logical' problem which Dr. Broad has generated about the different appearances which physical objects present when viewed under various conditions and from different distances and angles is a real problem; and also whether or not the Multiple Inherence Theory and the Multiple Relation Theory of Appearing are really contrary and alternative to common sense.

Dr. Broad exaggerates, I believe, the extent to which these two theories differ from common sense. Both theories allow that the objective constituents of visual situations may be 'literally spatio-temporal parts' of physical objects. But the Multiple Inherence Theory can allow this, he tells us, only by holding that the physical object can be both constant and variable in its spatial (and qualitative) characteristics within the same stretch of time. Now if the Multiple Inherence Theory did actually propose this,

[1] *Idem*, pp. 179 f.

it is obvious that it would not only be 'contrary to common sense', but wholly nonsensical. But it soon becomes evident from Dr. Broad's explanation that the Multiple Inherence Theory does not propose this in any straightforward sense. What the theory actually does propose is rather that specification of the spatial and qualitative characteristics of any object involves an essential reference to the place from which the object is perceived.

But now, is this really contrary to common sense? While I do not suppose that many common-sense observers are so fully aware of such facts as Dr. Broad is, I think it is certainly true that everyone, at some time or another, has realized that an object looks different under different conditions and from different distances and angles. Surely everyone is aware that an object seems to grow larger as it approaches, and smaller as it recedes, and that parallel lines seem to converge in the distance. Likewise, everyone knows that colour perception and colour phenomena as a whole are affected by lighting conditions, angle of reflection, contrast, distances, and various other subjective as well as objective factors. In everyday life we take account of such factors when we modify our judgments in such fashion as, for example: 'It looks square *from here*', or 'It looks green *in this light*'.

What, then, exactly, is the difference between the Multiple Inherence Theory and the common-sense view? It is, I believe, primarily, if not entirely, a verbal one. This becomes apparent when we ask ourselves what it is that we are led to expect by the Multiple Inherence Theory that we do not already expect on the common-sense view? Obviously the Multiple Inherence Theory is but a verbal rendering of the fact, already familiar to common sense, that it makes a difference where you stand when you try to judge the spatial and qualitative characteristics of objects visually. The explanation of this fact is, of course, to be found in physics and physiological psychology; and it is not contrary to common sense. The Multiple Inherence Theory, however, is clearly not an explanation at all. It is not even an *ad hoc* hypothesis. For an *ad hoc* hypothesis at least invents or invokes a distinct entity or process which will account for a given phenomenon; while the Multiple Inherence Theory merely legislates the alleged problem out of existence. In effect, it merely *allows* that the qualitities of physical objects may appear differently to different observers at the same time, and that they may appear differently to the same observer from different vantage points. It does not say anything about such qualities and spatial character- istics as colour, shape, and size except that this is true of them. But this was precisely the fact with which we started! The further postulate that objects *cannot* be described with respect to these predicates without a specification of the place of the observer is but a concession to verbal consistency. For the theory also allows the familiar fact that the visual qualities of an object may often appear the same from many different places, either for one and the same observer, or for different observers at once. (In those cases where an object reveals its actual colour, the distinction between sensible and physical is clearly artificial. In such instances it is purely a matter of choice of linguistic convention whether one is to say that the quality 'inheres dyadically', or, even so, 'triadically'.)

The language of the Multiple Inherence Theory, however, has the defect of obscuring the familiarity of the facts with which it deals. The statement that red, for example, is a characteristic such that it can only 'inhere in a place from a place' refers only to the familiar fact that the position of the observer makes a difference in the colour or the shade of colour an object will appear to him to have. But it suggests quite a different situation, wholly novel and exciting. The essence of the Multiple Inherence Theory, Dr. Broad tells us, is the distinction between the 'sensible' and the 'physical' inherence of a colour in a place. The former is the 'fundamental and indefinable' relation; and it is 'irreducibly triadic', involving an essential reference to the pervading shade of colour, the pervaded region, and the 'region of projection'. The latter, he says, is a two-term relation; but it is not ultimate, for it is definable in terms of the former. Now, of course, to predicate any quality or spatial characteristic of any object is, ultimately, to say something about its sensible effects; for language is, after all, a medium of communication about experience, in which the colours, shapes, and sizes of objects are elements. In this sense, everything may be said to be 'sensible': rocks and chairs and tables, as well as after-images and hallucinatory pink rats. Denying the distinction between physical and sensible, however, suggests something altogether different. It seems to obliterate the distinction between an object's actually being red, for instance, and its only appearing to be red—a distinction which we often have good ground for making. It suggests some mysterious unseen physical process by which objects are wiped clean of their colour (or lose their shapes!) when we turn our backs or shut our eyes. Or else it suggests that objects are not themselves coloured, but that we project the colour upon the surfaces of objects when we look at them, as though our gaze were like a coloured spotlight. And this obviously won't do. It makes a mystery of so much of everyday experience. If objects are not themselves coloured, it becomes a puzzle as to why, when we get a spot of red paint on our hands, for instance, and do not look at it again until some time later, it should still be red, and not some other colour; and why the perceptual judgments of others should agree with ours; and why colour photographs taken of objects when no one is looking at them should coincide with our experience when we do later look at the objects themselves; and so forth and so on. Obviously in all such cases there is some persistent physical characteristic in the object itself which is responsible for its consistently giving rise to the same colour experience. It is this *permanent disposition* which we have in mind when we say that colour is a physical property of objects themselves, and not *merely* a quality of sensation. Colour-blind individuals do not perceive the colour of objects, to be sure; but it no more follows from this, as I have previously had occasion to point out, that those who do perceive colour *project* it upon objects, than it follows from the fact that blind people do not see objects at all, that those who do see them *create* them in perception.

But, of course, the Multiple Inherence Theory is not a physical theory; and if it suggests these situations, it does so misleadingly. If it did actually assert something empirical about the properties of objects, the issue could soon be determined; minus these pragmatic connotations, however, it is semantically indistinguishable from the common-sense view.

The upshot is this. The Multiple Inherence Theory does rest upon a certain set of facts involving the relevance of the observer and his position, etc., to the perception of the characteristics of objects. But ordinary common-sense usage naturally and implicitly embraces these facts. The attempt to re-word common usage to take explicit cognizance of them only leads to confusion. For such language as Dr. Broad wants to employ in doing this ordinarily expresses states of affairs which are quite different from the familiar veridical perceptual situations of everyday life, and its use in such cases is either altogether unintelligible or else wholly misleading. In the ordinary sense in which such an assertion is made, it is perfectly correct to say, for example, that a given object is *actually* red, and does not *merely* appear to be so; and in this sense an assertion to the contrary would simply be false.

4

Let us consider now the Multiple Relation Theory of Appearing. This theory, too, allows that the objective constituents of visual situations may be 'literally spatio-temporal parts' of physical objects. And it allows, according to Dr. Broad, that '*if* the objective constituent did have such characteristics as it seems to have, they *would* inhere in it in the ordinary dyadic way which common-sense recognizes'. It can allow this, however, Dr. Broad insists, only by assuming that most, if not all, of the determinate characteristics which the objective constituent seems on careful inspection to have do not in fact inhere in it. It has to assume that the objective constituent of a visual situation can seem to 'appear' from a place to have characteristics which are other than and incompatible with the characteristics which it does have.

Now it seems to me that there is even less reason for holding this theory to be contrary and alternative to common sense than there was in the case of the Multiple Inherence Theory. As I have already observed, it is a matter of common knowledge that objects do present different appearances from different places and under different conditions. And in specifying these different appearances, the reference must obviously be triadic. I do not believe that the common-sense view that objects are literally or, in Dr. Broad's terminology, 'dyadically', coloured, or that they have a determinate physical shape and size, in any way intends to deny this fact. Hence, it is clear that there is not even a verbal difference between this 'theory' and the common-sense view.

Dr. Broad's language *about* this theory, however, again tends to obscure the familiarity of the facts with which it deals. For example, Dr. Broad writes that the Multiple Relation Theory of Appearing 'assumes a fundamental, unique and not further analysable relation of "appearing" between an object, my mind, and a given qualitative or spatial characteristic.[1] But I do not see that there is an 'assumption' at all involved in the view that objects appear to have characteristics other than those which they have in fact. For it is obviously a matter of empirical fact that this is often the case. The use of the term 'appear' involves us in no special 'theory' about perception, but is merely an arbitrary word-sign to denote an ostensible fact of experience. There can be no legitimate objection, I suppose, to the logical description of 'to appear' as a 'relation'. And it may also, as such, be described as a 'triadic' one involving an object, a mind, and a given predicate. But Dr. Broad's reference to the 'assumption of a fundamental, unique and not further analysable relation' seems to make a mystery of what is patently obvious and familiar. There is a perfectly adequate explanation of the fact that objects present different appearances under different conditions and from different distances and angles, to be found in optics, the principles of perspective, and the like, and in physiological psychology. This is not to say that our knowledge of these matters is complete, of course, but rather that these are the lines we must pursue if it is indeed an explanation we are seeking, and not a mere linguistic revision.

Dr. Broad, however, thinks that this 'theory' presents an insurmountable difficulty. On this theory, he tells us,

we may be acquainted in a perceptual situation with a spatio-temporal part of a certain physical object which we are said to be perceiving. But we learn only about the characteristics which it *seems* to have; and the more carefully we inspect the objective constituent the more we learn of its *apparent* properties only. And it is certain that it either does not actually *have* properties of this kind at all; or that, if it does, the apparent and the real properties can be identical only in one specially favoured perceptual situation. And there is of course nothing in any particular perceptual situation, taken by itself, to tell us that in it and it alone the apparent and the real characteristics of the objective constituent are identical.[2]

---

[1] *Idem*, p. 178. Cf. *Scientific Thought*, p. 237: 'The essential point . . . about theories of this kind is that they do not imply that we are aware of *anything* that *really is* elliptical when we have the experience which we express by saying that the penny looks elliptical to us. Theories of this type have been suggested lately by Professor Dawes Hicks and by Dr. G. E. Moore. So far, they have not been worked out in any great detail, but they undoubtedly deserve careful attention.'

[2] *The Mind and Its Place in Nature*, p. 179.

With respect to this objection, it is far from clear why Dr. Broad should even suggest as an alternative that the object 'does not actually *have* properties of this kind at all'—i.e., that it may not have *any* of the properties which it appears to have. If it be allowed, as the Multiple Relation Theory supposedly does, that the objective constituent of a perceptual situation can actually be a spatio-temporal part of the object which we are perceiving, then it seems to me that, provided our inspection is careful and thorough, the object *must* have at least *some* of the characteristics which it appears to have. The reason is twofold. In the first place, if we do inspect the object more and more carefully, then it seems clear that we are bound to arrive at the ideal conditions (i.e., normal lighting, rectangular perspective, etc.) which will enable us to get an accurate perceptual knowledge of its true properties. Only if our inspection is too cursory, it seems to me, is it empirically possible that the object should not have *any* of the properties which it appears to have. The second reason is a logical one. In order to ascertain that any property or set of properties did not truly characterize an object, it is obvious that we should have to know what properties *did* truly characterize the object. It is possible, of course, that none of *any given set* of properties characterize the object in question; but it is not logically possible that *all* the apparent properties should fail in this respect. For in that case it is not merely a practical matter of being unable to *ascertain* that the properties do not characterize the object. Rather the assertion that they do not is then robbed of all possible significance.

The argument that we can learn only about the characteristics which the object *seems* to have, and that there is nothing in any particular perceptual situation, taken by itself, to tell us that in it and it alone the apparent and the real characteristics of the objective constituent are identical, is a familiar one with Dr. Broad. We have already met and answered it, in a slightly different context. In raising this objection, I may again point out, Dr. Broad clearly misses the very point of the distinction between such terms as 'apparent' and 'real'. These terms are logically *polar* with respect to each other; and hence neither has any meaning without the other.

In holding that we learn through perception only about the characteristics which objects *seem* to have, Dr. Broad would appear to be labouring the tautology that 'all seen things are seen'. If 'appearance' be taken to mean any content of a perceptual situation, it is, of course, inescapable that we see appearances. After all, objects are perceived through the senses. But it does not follow from this that we see *mere* appearances. For in this sense 'appearance' is not a pejorative term. If it be granted that at least sometimes the objective constituent of our perceptual experience is literally a spatio-temporal part of an external physical object, then it follows that in those cases we *are* acquainted with the characteristics which the object *really* has. But even in these cases of veridical perception it would still be correct to say that we are acquainted with the *appearance* of the object; only then it is the *true* appearance. Ordinarily we distinguish between a *mere* appearance and reality. Thus we say that railroad tracks *merely appear* to converge in the distance, but that *in reality* they are parallel; or we say that a certain object *merely appears* to be yellow, because we are suffering from the effects of jaundice, and that *in reality* it is white. The distinction, however, is plainly a relative one. For by 'in reality' we don't mean to refer to some 'transcendent' realm of unperceivable and unknowable 'things-in-themselves'; rather we mean that which we do or can perceive and know under more reliable conditions; that which will square with the rest of our perceptual experience and knowledge. It is merely a verbal problem, then, which Dr. Broad raises in objecting that we can learn only the apparent properties of objects.

The proper question is not *whether* a distinction can be made between mere appearance and reality, but rather *on what basis* this distinction is to be made. Dr. Broad holds that the apparent and the real properties of objects can be identical only in one specially favoured perceptual situation, and he insists that there is nothing in any particular perceptual situation, taken by itself, to tell us that in it, and it alone, the apparent and the real characteristics are identical.

Now we have also encountered this objection before in Dr. Broad's argument; and the answer is again the same. In everyday life we recognize and make allowances for the effect of such conditions as lighting, distance, and perspective on our judgments respecting the colour, size, and shape of objects. But we are also aware that there are more or less 'normal' conditions, under which we can make judgments which will stand up under subsequent observation, in varying situations. There is, it must be admitted, no single concise rule-of-thumb which enables us to decide in all cases as to whether our judgments are veridical or not. Rather, each case, or at least each type of case, must be decided in terms of its own peculiar circumstances. For example, we know that if a certain object which appears to be yellow were really yellow, and did not merely look so because it was being viewed under a yellow spotlight, then shining blue light on it in an otherwise dark room would cause it to look green, and not blue, or etc. If necessary, we could perform this experiment; though usually it is sufficient, in cases of doubt, merely to view the object in ordinary daylight, or even under ordinary artificial lighting. In this way we would be able to determine the colour characteristic of the object itself, and to predict in a verifiable manner how it would look under various conditions.

Again, with respect to the geometric properties of objects, if what we are seeing from an oblique perspective is square, and not, as it might appear, oblong or diamond-shaped, its diagonals will be found upon measurement to be of equal length; and as we walk around it, its appearance will vary in a different way from that in which it would if it were really oblong or diamond-shaped. But there is no need to multiply instances. There clearly *are* ways of telling which are the true characteristics of objects.

5

In the light of the foregoing, I want to consider anew Dr. Broad's problem of the different appearances which the circular penny presents when viewed from various distances and perspectives. Now at the outset I want to point out that the kind of phenomenon to which Dr. Broad is here alluding is one with which everyone is perfectly familiar, what Dr. Broad says to the contrary, notwithstanding. It is a fact, he writes, that it often needs a good deal of persuasion to make a man believe that, when he looks at a penny from the side, it seems elliptical to him.[1] This, however, is not the sort of familiarity I have in mind. I do not mean to suggest that we have a ready knowledge of the exact degree of ellipticity, for example, which we expect of an actually round penny from any specifiable angle of observation.

[1] *Scientific Thought*, p. 246.

Nor do I mean that everyone, necessarily, is specifically conscious of the fact that objects do appear to have different geometric shapes from different points of observation. The point is rather that we do in fact achieve through experience a kind of inexplicit familiarity with the principles of perspective which enables us to expect and, especially, to *recognize* the proper degree of apparent geometric variation which objects present from various angles and distances of inspection. It is this inexplicit familiarity which enables even the merest layman to criticize the inexpert attempts at linear perspective of, say, the fourteenth-century Florentine painters. And it is the same familiarity which enables us to judge in advance the shape that an object which we have seen only from a distance will be found to have upon closer, more careful inspection.

This being granted, I want to raise two points with respect to Dr. Broad's assertion that 'there is nothing in any particular perceptual situation, taken by itself, to tell us that in it, and it alone, the apparent and the real characteristics are identical'.

I want to call attention, in the first place, to the words 'any particular situation, *taken by itself*'. Dr. Broad employed this device, it will be recalled, in arguing that because the 'external reference' of perceptual situations is sometimes false (e.g., in hallucinations), and because these situations 'differ in no relevant *internal* respect' from those in which the claim to 'external reference' is true, the claim that the objective constituent of a perceptual situation is in fact literally part of a larger external object cannot be accepted at its face-value. I want to reply to this argument again.

In introducing the Multiple Relation Theory of Appearing, Dr. Broad told us that while this theory allows that the objective constituent may sometimes be literally a spatio-temporal part of the object which we are seeing, it can do this only by assuming that the objective constituents of some perceptual situations have certain qualities which differ from and are inconsistent with those which they seem *on careful inspection* to have. I want to consider the phrase 'on careful inspection' in connection with the earlier phrase to which I have called attention, namely: 'any particular situation *taken by itself*'. Now if the objective constituent of the perceptual situation in which one is observing the penny from an oblique perspective is understood to be literally the visible part of the surface of the penny (which the Multiple

Relation Theory is supposed to admit), then it follows that a 'careful inspection' of the objective constituent means a careful inspection of the visible surface of the penny, and not a careful inspection of a single view of it, regarded as though it were an entity separate and distinct from any other view of the penny, like a photographic image. A careful inspection of the surface of the penny itself, it is clear, could not justifiably be limited to the single original perspective from which we first happened to see it. One would have to approach closely, handle it, and look at it from various angles, especially head-on, before he could be said to have made a 'careful inspection'. In that case, however, it would not be true that the 'objective constituent'—i.e., the penny—had characteristics different from and incompatible with those which it seemed *on careful inspection* to have. For careful inspection would reveal that the penny was actually round. In fact, the observer *could not* find that the penny had characteristics other than it seemed on careful inspection to have; for how else could he determine what characteristics the penny actually had, save by careful inspection? What other meaning can be given to the words: 'the characteristics which the penny actually has'?

It is clearly an artificial restriction which Dr. Broad imposes when he defies us to determine from a single perceptual situation, 'taken by itself', that in it 'the apparent and the real characteristics of the objective constituent are identical'. But this, however, is not to say that we can *never* tell in a given perceptual situation that our judgment is veridical, without further observations. Before me, as I write, is a penny. The penny looks circular to me from where I sit, and I know that my perception is correct. For I have examined this particular penny before; and, what is more important, I am seeing it now under more or less ideal conditions: from relatively close by, head-on, and under a good light. If I were called upon to justify my judgment, I could, I am certain, make a convincing case for it. But in doing so I would be convincing my challenger, and not myself. For my present perceptual situation is much too typical to justify my having any reasonable doubts. Moreover, we all see objects for the *first* time, and know at once that our judgments about them are accurate; because the perceptual situation in which we are seeing them is of a familiar and 'normal' kind. Of course, even in such cases it may be argued that it is not the particular perceptual situation 'taken by itself' which enables us to judge that the real and not *merely* the apparent characteristics of the object are being revealed to us. But this is obviously to win the case by defining the 'perceptual situation' in such a way as to insure against any possible refutation. On this extreme atomistic conception of experience, there is literally nothing that we could *know*. The very distinction between real and apparent, it is particularly important to note, could not be formulated on the basis of a single perception taken by itself. There would be nothing relevant to which it could be compared; and hence there would be no question as to whether it was true or false. Dr. Broad would then have no ground for raising his problem in the first place.

6

This brings me to the second of the two points which I want to raise concerning the difficulty which Dr. Broad finds in the Multiple Relation Theory. Dr. Broad argues that if we wish to keep both the common-sense notion of physical objects and the claim that the objective constituents of at least some perceptual situations are literally spatio-temporal parts of physical objects, we must hold that the objective constituents of these visual situations can have qualities which are different from and inconsistent with those which they seem on careful inspection to have. And he argues further that if the objective constituent does have any of the properties which it seems to have, the apparent and the real properties can be identical only in one specially favoured perceptual situation. Now I believe that Dr. Broad has exaggerated both in the extent to which he claims that the various appearances of an object differ from and are inconsistent with each other, and in limiting the identity of the apparent and real properties of an object to a single favoured situation.

In speaking of 'one specially favoured perceptual situation', Dr. Broad seems to be suggesting that only when one places his eyes just so many inches away from an object, at one precise angle of perspective, and in light of precisely one particular wavelength frequency and brightness, etc., etc., are the *real* characteristics of a given object revealed. Now if this were indeed the case, there might be some justification for the objection that it is extremely arbitrary to claim that only in one particular perceptual situation the 'true' characteristics of an object are revealed, all others revealing merely apparent characteristics. There would certainly be a question as to just how this particular situation was ascertained to be *the* right one. But of course the situation is nothing like this. It is usually not difficult for several people from different positions to make identical and accurate judgments as to the true colour, shape, or other characteristics of an object which they are simultaneously observing. Nor is it unusual for people who see a given object at different times and under fairly wide differences in light conditions, etc., to agree in their perceptual judgments about it.

Once more taking up the penny before me on the desk, and rotating it about close to the lamp, I find that it does, admittedly, vary in its appearance with respect to colour and shape. But I also find that through a considerable area of change in distance from my eyes, proximity to the lamp, and angle of perspective, I have no difficulty whatsoever in distinguishing the true shape and colour of the penny. It is only when I hold the penny a considerable distance from my eyes and close to the lamp at such an angle that it catches and reflects the light into my eyes, that I find any difficulty in distinguishing its natural colour. And it is only when I hold the flat surface of the penny at almost a full 180-degree angle in my line of sight that I must confess to experiencing difficulty in distinguishing its true shape. Thus, it is clear that Dr. Broad exaggerates when he says that it is only in one specially favoured perceptual situation that the apparent characteristics of the objective constituent coincide with its real characteristics, and can be ascertained.

Dr. Broad, however, might insist that in many of the situations from which I claim to be able to distinguish the true characteristics of the penny, more careful inspection of the objective constituent from the given position of observation would reveal it to have characteristics actually different from those which I attribute to the penny itself. Now there is a certain justification for this claim. As I rotate the penny before me, it makes different angles with respect to the lamp, and as a consequence there is subtle play of light and shadow on its surface which affects its apparent colour or shade of colour. But I do not think that this in any way constitutes a difficulty. The fact is that though the penny under these conditions does reveal characteristics which are not intrinsic to it, nevertheless this kind of change of appearance is not at all *incompatible* with what I attribute to the penny itself. Though I attribute a certain brownish natural copper colour to the penny, I also attribute a certain degree of polish to its surface. And I know that the variations in the qualitative appearance of the surface of the penny are due to the light from the lamp nearby, which is reflected differently by different portions of the surface of the penny, and not to any relevant intrinsic variation in the physical characteristics of the penny itself. For I find that if I hold the penny still, but move my hand about in such a way as to alter the reflection of light upon the penny's surface, I can affect and control at will the qualitative changes in its appearance. Thus I have no difficulty in identifying what I see to be the surface of the penny. I see it the way I do because that is the appearance which the penny itself presents to me, due to its property of reflecting light. What I see, the way the penny appears to me, is more or less exactly what would be reproduced by a photograph of the penny taken from the same position. Thus, at least with respect to colour, I have shown that Dr. Broad is mistaken in holding that the apparent characteristics of the object are inconsistent with its true characteristics save in one specially favoured perceptual situation.

Perhaps Dr. Broad would concede the foregoing, however, but would insist that I have neglected to mention the apparent changes in the *shape* of the penny as I observe it from various angles. He would insist, I think, that at any other than a rectangular perspective, careful inspection of the objective constituent would reveal it to be elliptical in appearance, and not round. Now the fact is that I do not want to deny this, either; and yet, again, I think that this admission is not at all incompatible either with the assertion that the objective constituent of the various visual situations in which this is true is literally a spatio-temporal part of the penny which is actually round, nor with my earlier assertion that even in these situations the objective constituent looks round and not elliptical. I want to try to show this.

Suppose an elliptical disc were viewed first head-on and then from an oblique perspective. In that case there is no question but that the object would be seen and judged to look elliptical from either and both perspectives. And both judgments would be correct in the usual sense of the words 'look elliptical.' But now, when it is said of a *round* penny that it looks elliptical, I want to suggest that it is open to question whether the words 'looks elliptical' are being used in their ordinary sense. It is with this point in mind, I believe, that some to whom the distinctive appearance of a penny when viewed obliquely has been specifically pointed out, have still insisted that the penny viewed in this way looks round, and not elliptical. Actually there is good ground for this insistence. For the truth is that the round penny looked at in this way does not actually look as though it were elliptical, but rather it looks, as Professor G. E. Moore has put it, *like* an ellipse, *only with something peculiar about it*. And this peculiarity, I venture to say, is that its surface 'looks elliptical' only to the familiar degree and in the familiar way that we expect an actually round penny to look when viewed from that general position, and it does not look either the way the surface of an elliptical disc of that degree of eccentricity ought to look when viewed from that distance and perspective, or even the way it looks when viewed head-on.

The phrase 'looks elliptical' is ambiguous in two respects. In the first place, there is an ambiguity in that it may be taken to mean, on the one hand, that the penny 'looks as though it were actually elliptical'; and on the other, only that it 'looks like an ellipse looks'. In the former sense, of course, it is not true that the round penny viewed obliquely 'looks elliptical'. For the penny looks like a round object ought to look when viewed in that way. It looks as though it were actually round, and not as though it were actually elliptical. But now, again, there is a further ambiguity even in the case of the second interpretation: 'looks like an ellipse looks'. For this phrase, as it stands, is incomplete. As I have already pointed out, it is a perfectly familiar and common-sense fact that the way an object looks depends on the place from which it is being seen. Thus, if the phrase is to be made complete, we must specify the *place* from which the appearance is being described. We must, for example, distinguish between 'looking the way an ellipse would look from the same distance and angle', and 'looking the way an ellipse would look from close by and head-on'. Now obviously it is only in the second sense that a penny viewed from the side and at a distance can properly be said—if at all—to 'look elliptical'. (Again, some would insist, justifiably, I believe, that the penny looked at from the side does not look properly like an actually elliptical surface viewed either obliquely or rectangularly.) In any event, this sense in which the penny 'looks elliptical' is not at all incompatible with its being round and looking so from a rectangular perspective. And it is on this claim that Dr. Broad bases his objection to the identification of the objective constituent as a literal spatio-temporal part of the physical object.

From the foregoing, it should be clear that Dr. Broad is mistaken in holding that all the appearances of the penny save that which it presents from a direct, head-on view do not belong to the penny itself, but are rather, somehow, illusory. Let us consider, for example, the appearance which parallel railroad tracks present of converging off in the distance. That this phenomenon is properly called an 'illusion' is a verbal issue which I do not want to argue. But I do think that there is a very important difference between this type of 'illusion' and the kind of which the familiar Muller-Lyer Illusion is an example. In the latter, it will be recalled, we are confronted with two horizontal parallel lines of equal length. One of these lines is capped at either end by arrow heads in such a way as not to extend the over-all length of the line; the other is capped by an arrow tail at either end, extending the over-all length of the figure to form a kind of letter 'Y' with each end of the line. The illusion consists in the fact that the original horizontal line of the figure capped with the arrow tails, though measurably exactly the same length as the original horizontal line of the figure capped with the arrow heads, looks to be longer. Now even in this illusion, to be sure, we do not have a case of the objective constituent actually appearing on careful inspection to have properties different from those which it is actually supposed to have, but rather only a case of the two lines which comprise the objective constituent being mistakenly *judged* to be of unequal length. For if we examine the objective constituent carefully enough, we shall be able to ascertain that the lines are actually of equal length. The illusion arises, I believe, from the difficulty we have in excluding the irrelevant figures at the end of each line from our attention and judgment. Be this as it may, however, there is a sense in which it may be said that the objective constituent 'appears' (i.e., on first uncritical inspection) to have a characteristic different from and inconsistent with that which we actually attribute to the lines themselves. And the point which I want to make is this: even if we did not succeed in detecting the equality of the lines which comprise the objective constituent, by direct inspection alone, if the two figures were to be photographed together (from the same position as our eyes), and the photograph were to be superimposed on lined graph paper, it would become apparent at once that the stimuli reaching our eyes from the two lines were actually of equal length.

Let us consider, now, what we would find it we photographed the apparently converging railroad tracks in the same way. The fact is that the outline of the image which the tracks would form on the photographic film superimposed on the lined graph paper would plainly be, not parallel, but converging. Now this is obviously not a case of the objective constituent being *judged* to have characteristics other than it actually has; neither is it a case of the objective constituent *appearing* to have properties which are different from and inconsistent with those which it really has. The way the tracks appear to us is the way they are actually presented to our eyes. But how, then, is this fact to be reconciled with the further fact that the tracks themselves are supposed to be *actually* parallel, if we are to maintain the view that the objective constituent is literally a spatio-temporal part of the object—the tracks—itself? The answer, I believe, is obvious enough. The tracks *are* actually parallel. They were laid so as to be parallel, and nothing has occurred to alter their gauge. The point is simply that we are seeing them from a distance; and because of the nature of the human eye, and the behaviour of light by means of which we see objects, our perception of them, their appearance to us, obeys the perfectly understandable principles of optical perspective.

Applying these considerations, now, to the case of seeing the penny from an oblique angle, I want to point out that here too what we see is what is presented to our eyes. A photograph of the penny taken from the same position and super-imposed as before upon lined graph paper would show that the impression which the light reflected from the penny makes upon the retina of the eye was actually elliptical in outline. Thus, this too is not a case of the objective constituent appearing to have characteristics different from and incompatible with those which it actually has;

nor, again, is it a case of the objective constituent not being literally a spatio-temporal part of the object. The objective constituent of my perception is the surface of the circular penny itself; but it is the surface of the circular penny as it can be seen from an oblique angle, with all the limitations imposed by the nature of the human eye and the behaviour of light. And this fully and understandably accounts for the distinctive appearances. The limitations are overcome, of course, when we look directly down upon the penny. It is then that we see what we call its 'true shape', undistorted by perspective. To hold that this is its 'true shape', however, is not a whimsical or arbitrary legislation, as Dr. Broad suggests. For it is the shape which is corroborated by tactual inspection and physical measurement, and which, alone, will account for the various successive appearances of the penny as it is observed from different distances and angles.

Thus we see that the various appearances of the penny, though different, are not, as Dr. Broad holds, *inconsistent*, either with each other or with the actual shape of the penny. They are perfectly consistent in view of the nature of light, the principles of geometric perspective, and the nature of the human eye. Quite the contrary, what *would* be inconsistent, in view of these facts, would be for the penny to present the same appearance regardless of the distance and angle from which it is inspected!

7

Finally, I want to point out that Dr. Broad would not consider that his problem has been solved by the foregoing comments. Witness the following passage:

It is probable that at first sight the reader will not see much difficulty in this. He will be inclined to say that we can explain these various visual appearances by the laws of perspective and so on. This is not a relevant answer. It is quite true that we can *predict what particular appearance* an object will present to an observer, when we know the shape of the object and its position with respect to the observer. But this is not the question that is troubling us at present. Our question is as to the compatibility of these changing elliptical appearances, however they may be correlated with other facts in the world, with the supposed constancy and roundness of the physical object.[1]

[1] *Idem*, pp. 235 f.

It would seem that Dr. Broad is determined to have his problem! To these remarks I can only reply that, far from being *irrelevant*, it is perfectly obvious that the laws of perspective resulting from the behaviour of light and the nature of the human eye offer the *only relevant* answer. They show *why* the penny presents the different appearances it does from different points of observation, and they also thus show how these different appearances are compatible one with another and with the actual shape of the penny. It is not, however, merely a matter of predicting what particular appearance an object will present to an observer from different points of observation; rather it is a matter of understanding the physical and psycho-physiological processes involved in seeing. We do not learn simply by rote the specific degree-by-degree variations in the way objects appear to us as we move about. If this were the case, it should not surprise us at all if, say, in observing the receding parallel rails from the back of a moving railroad train, we found that they appeared to *converge* up to a certain point in the distance, but then suddenly appeared to *diverge* beyond that point. Such a phenomenon would be beyond our comprehension in a way which the actual familiar phenomena of visual perspective are not. We should simply have to accept it as a brute contingent fact. But in view of the known facts, we certainly should be incredulous if we were to have such an experience; and we should suspect that the rails had been mechanically altered in some way after we had passed over them, or that we were seeing them through some unusual refractive medium. This is because our knowledge of perspective is not, as Dr. Broad would have us believe, simply a matter of predicting appearances *a posteriori*, on the basis of exhaustive detailed observation, but stems rather from our theoretical insight and comprehension of the processes involved.

As I have shown, the changing appearances of the penny as we observe it from different positions are not only wholly compatible with the supposed constancy of the penny, and with its actual roundness as revealed from a head-on view, but are actually *demanded* by the behaviour of light and the nature of the eye. If the observer were standing still, and the penny which is supposed to have a constant shape appeared to change from round to elliptical, then there would indeed be a problem. It would be a problem to which the known principles of perspective would admittedly not be a sufficient answer. But when the observer is known to move about, why, obviously the principles according to which the light, by means of which he sees the penny, reaches his eyes will be relevant. To say that our knowledge of the principles of optics is irrelevant to the explanation of the phenomena we are considering is as absurd as it would be to say that Kepler's laws of planetary motion and the laws of gravitation and the like are not relevant explanations for the observable behaviour of planets, but are merely descriptions by means of which we are fortuitously able to make successful predictions!

CHAPTER V

THE 'CAUSAL QUESTION'

THE preceding chapter was concerned with the 'logical problem' which arises, according to Dr. Broad, when we try to maintain the common-sense view that the objective constituents of perceptual situations are literally spatio-temporal parts of external physical objects, in the face of apparently contradictory appearances. What this problem demanded, Dr. Broad held, was a reconsideration of the formal characteristics of the relation of such attributes as shape, size, and colour to the objective constituents of perceptual situations, and to physical objects. In this connection we examined and criticized Dr. Broad's answer to this demand in the form of the Theory of Multiple Inherence and the Multiple Relation Theory of Appearing, which he presented as alternatives to the common-sense view. In the present chapter I want to discuss the 'causal question' which Dr. Broad asks, and the answer which he presents.

I

The causal question which Dr. Broad wishes us to consider may be stated as follows: In view of what we know of geometrical and physical optics and of the physiology of vision,[1] what are the

---

[1] Interestingly enough, Dr. Broad does not hesitate to employ here just those causal considerations which, as we saw in the previous chapter, he dismisses as irrelevant to the problem which he raised concerning the discrepant appearances of objects from various perspectives. This seems to be a clear case of special pleading. It may be observed that the illegitimate use of specific knowledge which his own views either deny or render doubtful is a recurrent and disturbing difficulty throughout Dr. Broad's argument.

conditions under which such and such characteristics of the objective constituents of perceptual situations will be manifested; what are the 'independently necessary and sufficient conditions' for (say) a certain shade of colour to characterize the objective constituent of a particular perceptual situation, and where are these causal conditions located?[1] In answering this question, there are, according to Dr. Broad, three causal considerations which we must bear in mind. I shall present them briefly.

The first consideration involves complications in perception due to mirrors, non-homogeneous media, and the like.[2] When one looks at the reflection of a luminous point in a plane mirror, the region which is pervaded from where he is standing is somewhere behind the mirror. It is the place where a luminous point would have to be put in order to present the actual appearance, if viewed directly and without a mirror, from where one is standing. But, of course, nothing physically relevant is happening at this place behind the mirror. Now the direction of this place for the observer is determined by the direction in which the light enters his eyes; and its distance along this direction is presumably determined by traces left in the observer's brain by past visual situations and correlated bodily movements in cases where the vision really was direct and through a homogeneous medium. Hence, Dr. Broad argues, the pervasion of this place is determined by physical and psychological events in the immediate neighbourhood of the region of projection.[3]

Now of course, Dr. Broad observes, the physical events within the region of projection have physical causes. When a certain place is pervaded by very similar shades of the same colour from all directions, it is generally found, he tells us, that on walking up to this place, tactual situations arise whose objective constituents are closely correlated with the objective constituents of the successive visual situations which occur as we walk up to this place. We say then that this place is 'tactually occupied';

---

[1] *The Mind and Its Place in Nature*, p. 165.
[2] *Idem*, pp. 165 ff.
[3] It will be recalled, from the discussion of the Multiple Inherence Theory in the preceding chapter, that the term 'pervasion' refers to what, in ordinary language, would be called '*apparent* pervasion'; and that the pervasion of a place by a colour is described as a 'triadic relation' involving the pervading shade of colour, the pervaded region, and the 'region of projection' or place *from* which the pervaded region appears to contain the pervading shade of colour.

and we have very good reason to believe that such a region is physically occupied by 'certain microscopic events which are remote and dependently necessary conditions of the pervasion of this region by such and such a shade of colour from places around it'. These events, Dr. Broad says, determine by physical causation certain events in our eyes, optic nerves, and brains; and the latter events are the 'immediately necessary and sufficient material conditions of the pervasion of the external region by such a shade of colour from the region of projection which contains our bodies'. Thus, in the analysis of perceptual situations, we must, according to Dr. Broad, consider four factors: the pervaded region, the pervading shade of colour, and the region of projection, which comprise the triadic relation of sensible inherence; and, in addition, the 'emitting region', containing the microscopic physical events which determine by physical causation the events in our eyes, optic nerves, and brains, which in turn result in the apparent pervasion of a certain place by a certain shade of colour.

Most often, in everyday practical life, Dr. Broad acknowledges, the pervaded region and the emitting region roughly coincide. Such situations may be regarded as the normal case, he says; and they are expressed in common language by saying that we are then 'looking directly at a certain physical object through a colourless homogeneous medium'. But this 'sweet simplicity', though normal, is not universal, Dr. Broad points out. In the case of mirror-images and the visual situations which arise when we are surrounded by non-homogeneous media, the pervaded region and the emitting region cease to coincide, and may be very distant from each other. When a number of people 'see the same mirror-image', the physical events in the emitting region are, in fact, as far in front of the mirror as the pervaded region is behind it. The pervaded region may contain no physical events at all; or, if it does, they will be quite irrelevant.

The second of the three causal factors which Dr. Broad offers for our consideration has to do with the finite velocity of light. The facts which make us ascribe a velocity to light, and particularly the fact of aberration, make it almost certain, he argues, that the date at which a certain place is pervaded by a certain shade of colour from a certain region of projection is the date at which certain events are happening within the region of projection.

When we look at a distant star, a certain shade of colour sensibly inheres in a certain distant region from the place which is physically occupied by our bodies. But in view of the finite velocity of light, it may very well be that the star no longer physically occupies this distant region. And whether it does so or not, the relevant physical events may have happened there hundreds of years ago. Thus, corresponding to the distinction between the pervaded region and the emitting region, Dr. Broad contrasts the 'date of pervasion' and the 'date of emission'. Owing to the great velocity of light, these generally coincide almost exactly in the visual situations of ordinary life, just as ordinarily the pervaded region and the emitting region roughly coincide. Nevertheless, in the case of very remote objects such as the stars, the date of emission may precede the date of pervasion by thousands of years. And in any case, Dr. Broad insists, the date of emission is *always* earlier than the date of pervasion.[1]

Finally, as the third causal consideration, Dr. Broad asks us to consider such facts as colour-blindness and the effects of drugs like santonin and of morbid bodily states like jaundice. Such facts, he argues, make it practically certain that the particular colour and the particular shade which sensibly pervade an external place from a region of projection are determined by specific events in the eyes, optic nerves, and brain which physically occupy this region of projection at the time the external region is sensibly pervaded.[2]

In view of these considerations, then, what answer is implied for the causal question stated at the outset? Dr. Broad tells us that he thinks they show the following answer to be *almost* certain: 'The *independently* necessary and sufficient *material* conditions for a certain shade of colour to pervade a certain external region from a certain region of projection are all contained in or are close to the region of projection.'[3]

2

With this brief exposition of the causal considerations to which Dr. Broad calls our attention, and the answer which he thinks they imply for the causal question, I want to turn to the business

---

[1] *Idem*, pp. 166 f.   [2] *Idem*, p. 167.
[3] *Idem*, p. 165.

of criticism. Now at the conclusion of his exposition and defence of the Multiple Inherence Theory, Dr. Broad states that there are three points on which these causal considerations show common sense to be in error. Inasmuch as Dr. Broad contends that these considerations and their implications must be recognized by *any* satisfactory theory,[1] it is important to consider them carefully; and I propose to do this in terms of the three points on which Dr. Broad supposes that they contradict common sense.

Let us turn to the first point on which, according to Dr. Broad, common sense is in error.

(1) It believes that the colours which it sees are quite literally spread out over the surfaces of the *physical objects* which it sees and touches. In view of the facts about mirror-images, etc., we can admit only that colours pervade *regions of Space*. The latter may or may not contain those microscopic physical things and events which are the dependently necessary conditions of the pervasion of this region by this colour. Even when this is so, i.e., when there is an emitting as well as a pervaded region and the two coincide, we cannot say that the microscopic events and objects have the colour; we can say only that the region which contains them is pervaded by this colour.[2]

Now I do not find it at all clear why Dr. Broad should suppose that the fact that mirrors sometimes mislead us into judging that a certain place is occupied by an object of a certain colour, when in fact that place is not thus occupied, forces us to the conclusion that colours only 'pervade regions of space', and are not, as common sense is supposed to hold, 'literally spread out over the surfaces of physical objects'. But I think his argument may be something like this. Sometimes a coloured object may appear to be in a certain place when in fact we are merely seeing a mirror-image of it, and no such object exists in that place. Still, that region does *appear* to us to be pervaded by a certain patch of colour. Thus, it would seem that a given region may appear to contain (i.e., 'may be pervaded by') a certain colour even though there is no object in that place on which that colour is 'literally spread out'.

But now what about those cases in which we are seeing an object directly, without the complications arising from mirror-reflections and the like? Why cannot we say in such cases, where there is a physical object in the pervading region, that the colour

---

[1] *Idem*, p. 178. [2] *Idem*, pp. 174 f.

which we see *is* 'literally spread out' over the surface of the object? Again Dr. Broad's argument is not clear; but I think it may very likely be this. The 'sweet simplicity' of this, the *normal* case, is not universal. There often are mirrors and other complications, and we must be prepared to deal with the general case.[1] 'If we want to clear up the meaning of some commonly used concept it is enormously important to see how it applies to exceptional and abnormal cases.'[2] Now in theory we can either take the normal case as fundamental, and try to explain the abnormal case of the mirror-image by making a number of supplementary hypotheses; or we can take the more complex abnormal case as fundamental, and regard the simpler normal case as due to the fulfilment of certain special conditions which *need* not be realized but which in fact generally are. 'The latter seems to be the only hopeful course to take.' Thus, in view of all the specified complications, we conclude that the sensible inherence of a certain shade of colour in a certain place is fundamentally triadic, involving an indispensable reference to a region of projection; and that the physical inherence of a colour in a place is a derived notion, ultimately reducible to the notion of sensible inherence or 'pervasion of a region of Space'. And from this it follows that even when the region of space which is pervaded by a certain colour contains 'those microscopic physical things and events which are the dependently necessary conditions of the pervasion of this region by this colour . . . i.e., when there is an emitting region as well as a pervaded region and the two coincide, we cannot say that the microscopic events and objects have the colour; we can say only that the region which contains them is pervaded by the colour'.

There are, then, two arguments which we must consider: first, whether the fact of mirror-images justifies the inference that colours may only pervade regions of space; and secondly, whether the fact of abnormal cases justifies the conclusion that even in veridical cases the most that we can say is that colours pervade only regions of space, and are not literally 'spread out' over physical objects.

In reply to the first argument, I want to begin by pointing out

[1] Cf. *idem*, p. 166.
[2] C. D. Broad, 'Critical and Speculative Philosophy', in *Cont. Brit. Phil.* (First Series), J. H. Muirhead, ed., pp. 90 f. I am here employing Dr. Broad's argument for the 'Principle of Exceptional Cases' as it occurs in his contribution to this volume. (Cf. Introduction, *supra*.)

the obvious fact that when, owing to mirror reflection, a coloured object appears to be at a place where in actual fact no such object exists, what appears to be in that place is not merely a colour, but a *coloured object*. When I see the reflection of a rose in a mirror, for example, what appears to me to be behind the mirror, as it were, is not merely a vaporous patch of red colour, but a red rose whose colour is 'spread out over its surface' in the same apparent manner in which this is true when I see the rose directly. Of course, there is actually no such object at that place, when what I am seeing is merely a mirror reflection; but then neither is there actually such a colour there. There *appears* to be such a colour there, it is true; but then there also *appears* to be such an object there. It seems to me, therefore, that there is no more justification to be found in the phenomenon of mirror-reflection for saying that colours only pervade regions of space than there is for saying that objects only pervade regions of space. And in that case we may equally well say that *coloured objects* pervade regions of space, and that the colours appear to be spread out over the surfaces of the objects. So much for the argument that the existence of mirror-images justifies the assertion that colours which are not literally characteristics of physical objects can by themselves pervade regions of space. The existence of mirror-images, at least, offers no good reason for the adoption of this strange mode of speech.

We must bear in mind, however, that what Dr. Broad means by the term 'pervade' is what we should ordinarily express by some such qualification as '*appears*' to pervade, employing the term 'pervade' in a physical sense. Thus, if we were to grant even the proposition that 'we can say only that *coloured objects* pervade regions of space', we should really be acquiescing in the proposition that 'we can say only that coloured objects *appear* to occupy regions of space'. Now, of course, it is sometimes true— e.g., in the case of mirror reflections—that we can say only that a (particular) physical object *appears* to occupy a (particular) region of space. For a particular object may, due to the fact that it is seen in mirror reflection, appear to be located at a certain place behind the mirror, when in actual fact it is as far in front of the mirror as it appears to be behind it. But what Dr. Broad means, of course, is that the most we can *ever* say is only that colours *appear* to occupy regions of space; and hence our modified statement (substituting 'coloured objects' for 'colours)', to be equivalent, would have to mean that the most we can *ever* say is only that coloured objects *appear* to occupy regions of space—i.e., but don't 'really' do so. And this is certainly false; for there are normal cases.

This brings us to the second argument. By Dr. Broad's Principle of Exceptional Cases, physical inherence, as we saw in the preceding chapter, is 'reduced' to sensible inherence. But I also showed there that this reduction is either merely verbal, or else it does violence to the facts which underlie the common-sense distinction between *mere* appearance and physical actuality. Just as there obviously is a distinction between a white object only appearing to be red because it is seen under red light, and an object which is actually red, so there is certainly a real distinction between an object only appearing to be in a certain place, for whatever reason, and an object actually being in that place.

That Dr. Broad is himself fully aware of the existence of such a distinction, moreover, is evident from the very arguments which he offers in denying it. The facts of jaundice, santonin, and the like are relevant only because they show that appearances are sometimes deceptive. Obviously Dr. Broad can recognize them *as* deceptive only because he does know what is *actually* the case in those situations in which such factors militate against accurate perception, as opposed to what only appears to be the case. And this is clearly true of his reference to mirror-images. For he explicitly shows that he knows what is actually the case, when he points out that when we see an object reflected in the mirror, 'it is in fact as far in front of the mirror as the pervaded region is behind it'.[1]

Now sometimes, it is true, we are not aware that what we are seeing is only a mirror reflection; and we judge that the object which we see in this way actually is where it appears to be.[2] But

[1] *The Mind and Its Place in Nature*, p. 168.

[2] It is time to point out that there is also a sense in which it may properly be said that objects which we see reflected in mirrors *appear to be where they actually are*. For if we are acquainted with the properties of mirrors, and know that we are seeing an object via mirror reflection, we are able to judge correctly as to the actual location of the object. Thus, when one looks in a mirror, he may see the reflection of a window which *appears to be* behind him; and when he turns around he sees that the window actually is where it appeared to be—behind him. It must be remembered that our ability to judge visual distance and location is, in *any* case, learned through experience. Our knowledge of the reflective behaviour of mirrors and of the effects of non-homogeneous media is a part of that experience.

this need occasion no difficulty. We have simply made a mistake, which we can discover if we inspect the situation more carefully. The fact that mirror reflections may cause us to judge that a certain region is occupied when it is in fact not occupied does not require us to adopt any change in our conception of physical objects as occupying space, or in our conception of colours as characteristics of objects. Dr. Broad, as I have pointed out, is perfectly familiar with the principles of mirror reflection, and with the fact that a reflected object is actually as far in front of the mirror as it illusorily appears to be behind it. And if he recognizes this difference between 'actually being' and 'illusorily appearing to be', then he is in substantial agreement with common sense as to the empirical facts.

Thus, I have refuted both aspects of Dr. Broad's first causal argument against common sense; and the gist of my arguments is this. In the case of mirror-images, describing the region behind the mirror, which appears to be occupied but actually is not, as being 'pervaded' by colour not only does not tell us any more about the facts than we already know, but it suggests something wholly misleading and mysterious. The fact of abnormal cases, on the other hand, does not justify the conclusion that even in normal cases the most we can say is that colours only pervade regions of space, and are not 'literally spread out over the surfaces of objects'. Application of this notion to the normal case via the Principle of Exceptional Cases is wholly gratuitous, and is nothing more than a suggestion for a new and quite unnecessary way of speaking about perfectly familiar facts.

3

The second point on which causal considerations show common sense to be in error, according to Dr. Broad, is as follows:

(2) Common-sense believes that the pervasion of anything by a colour is a two-term relation between this thing and this colour. In view of the fact that the whole top of the same penny may appear brown to me and yellow to you, who have taken santonin, we cannot admit this. If we wish to hold that this one surface really is the common constituent of your visual situation and mine, and that it really has the colours which it seems to you and me on careful inspection to have, we must hold that the sensible pervasion of a region by a colour is at

least a three-term relation. It must involve an essential reference to a region of projection as well as to the pervaded region and the pervading colour.[1]

Now I have already replied to this argument, in its essentials, in the discussion of Dr. Broad's 'logical question' in the preceding chapter. And I cannot see that the introduction of such causal considerations as the effects of santonin, jaundice, or other morbid bodily states materially affects the answer which I gave there. Hence I propose to leave this point without further discussion in order to turn to the new considerations which are presented in Dr. Broad's statement of the third point on which he alleges common sense to be in error.

4

Dr. Broad's third point of disagreement with common sense brings us to grips directly with the answer which he thinks the causal considerations noted above necessitate for the causal question; and it provides much material warranting careful analysis. I want to state this point in full in Dr. Broad's own words, and then to consider his argument in some detail, in the several sections which follow.

(3) Common-sense believes that the independently necessary and sufficient conditions for the pervasion of a certain region by a certain colour are contained in *that* region at the time when it is pervaded by this colour. It therefore holds that this region would be pervaded by this colour at this moment no matter what might be going on elsewhere. This cannot be accepted. The *independently* necessary and sufficient conditions for the pervasion of a certain region by a certain colour are *never* contained in the pervaded region and are *always* contained in or near the region of projection. It is true that, in favourable cases, the *dependently* necessary conditions for this pervasion may *have been* contained in the pervaded region; viz., when there is an emitting region and it coincides with the pervaded region. But, in the first place, there may be no emitting region at all. (Cf. the visual situations of dreams, or the case of the drunkard and his pink rats.) Secondly, there may be an emitting region, but it may be quite remote from the pervaded region. (Cf. mirror-images and aberration.) And lastly, even when there is an emitting region and it coincides with the pervaded region, common-sense is always wrong about the date of the relevant physical

[1] *The Mind and Its Place in Nature*, p. 175.

events in this region. It always assumes that they are contemporary with the pervasion, whereas they are always earlier and may be earlier by thousands of years.[1]

Now I want at the outset to clarify two points with respect to Dr. Broad's assertion that common sense holds that a certain region which is pervaded by a certain colour would be pervaded by this colour at this moment no matter what might be going on elsewhere. In the first place, as I have already pointed out, Dr. Broad's use of the term 'pervaded' stems from his argument that such characteristics as colour and shape do not literally characterize physical objects as such, but can only 'inhere-in-a-place-from-a-place'. The essence of the Multiple Inherence Theory (in terms of which Dr. Broad discusses the 'causal question'), it will be recalled, is the distinction between the 'sensible' and the 'physical' inherence of a quality in a place, and the claim that the latter is not ultimate, but is to be defined in terms of the former. The former, Dr. Broad told us, is the fundamental and indefinable relation; and it is 'irreducibly triadic', involving an essential reference to the pervading quality (e.g., shade of colour), the pervaded region, and the region of projection. The latter region refers to the locus of the observer, or place *from* which the pervaded region appears to contain the pervading quality. From all this it is clear that when Dr. Broad speaks of a certain region as being 'pervaded' by a certain shade of colour, he does not have in mind the common-sense proposition that there is actually present in that region something which has that shade of colour. Rather his use of the expression 'the region pervaded by a certain shade of colour' refers only to that fact which in ordinary language might be expressed as 'the region which *appears* to contain a certain shade of colour'.

It would seem, then, that Dr. Broad is asserting in this third point of disagreement that common sense would hold that a certain region could *appear* to contain a certain colour regardless of what might be going on elsewhere. Now if Dr. Broad *is* in fact using the term 'pervade' here in the sense which I have described, and hence *does* mean to assert this, then he is clearly in error as to the view which he attributes to common sense. For certainly it is a matter of common sense that unless someone were looking at and seeing a given place, that place would not appear either to

[1] *Idem*, pp. 175 f.

be occupied or not to be occupied; for in that case it couldn't properly be said to *appear* at all. Inasmuch as the 'region of projection' is by definition the place where the percipient individual is, it follows of necessity that an indispensable condition for any region to *appear* to be occupied is contained within the region of projection. And hence it would be contrary to common sense to hold that a given region could be 'pervaded', in this sense, by a certain colour, 'no matter what might be going on elsewhere'.

It may be, however, that Dr. Broad here means to employ the term 'pervade' in a *neutral* sense, so as to avoid the difficulty which I have just pointed out. It may be that he is employing the words 'the pervasion of a certain region by a certain colour' in an ambiguous sense, to mean simply the general, abstract notion of the presence of a colour in a place—whether perceived or not, and without begging the question of the proper analysis of the concept 'presence of a colour in a place'—in order to be able to reaffirm his point that a colour is a quality such that it can inhere only *sensibly* 'in-a-place-from-a-place', and to make the further assertion that the 'independently necessary and sufficient conditions' for the sensible inherence of a colour in a place are always contained in or near the region of projection.

Even if the term 'pervaded' is used in this general sense, however, it is still not true that common sense would hold that *whenever* a region is 'pervaded' by a certain colour, this region would be pervaded by this colour at this moment no matter what might be going on elsewhere. For common sense recognizes the existence of hallucinations, after-images, and the like; and it recognizes that when a certain region appears to be occupied by a certain colour, it may be that that appearance is purely hallucinatory. And in that case the 'presence' of colour in that region at that moment is not independent of what is going on elsewhere; for, quite the contrary, it is solely a function of the condition of the subject of that experience, who may be situated at a place quite remote from the region which appears to be occupied.

The second point of clarification which I want to make at the outset is this. It seems to me possible that the conclusions which Dr. Broad draws from the causal considerations which are the subject of this chapter are intended to follow only in conjunction with the 'logical argument' which we considered in the preceding chapter, that the pervasion of a certain region by a certain colour is a triadic relation and that the physical inherence of a colour in a place is reducible to the notion of sensible inherence. Thus, it may be that Dr. Broad's assertion that common sense is wrong in holding that the independently necessary and sufficient conditions for the pervasion of a certain region by a certain colour are contained in that region is not intended to be a *further* and independent attack on common sense, but is merely a causal consequence of his original 'logical' thesis. And in that case, I believe that I have already replied satisfactorily to Dr. Broad's 'logical argument', and, *a fortiori*, to this causal consequence.

Be this as it may, however, Dr. Broad does argue as though the causal considerations mentioned in this third point of disagreement with common sense constitute at least independent supporting reasons for both the 'logical' thesis that colours only pervade (i.e., 'sensibly and triadically inhere in') regions of space, and for the 'casual' thesis (or consequence) that the independently necessary and sufficient conditions for this to occur are contained in the region of projection. And since Dr. Broad insists that these causal considerations must be recognized by *any* satisfactory theory, I deem it necessary and worthwhile to consider them on their own merit. Hence, though I cannot agree that colour can *only* inhere sensibly and triadically 'in-a-place-from-a-place', I want to see to what extent, if any, we need grant even that the 'independently necessary and sufficient conditions' for the *sensible* pervasion of a certain region by a certain colour 'are *never* contained in the pervaded region and are *always* contained in the region of projection'.

5

With the preliminary comments out of the way, I want to begin the discussion of Dr. Broad's third point of disagreement with common sense with a comment on the initial implausibility of the contention that the independently necessary and sufficient conditions for the pervasion of a region by a certain colour are never contained in the pervaded region and are always contained in or near the region of projection. Dr. Broad has said that the direction of the pervaded region is the direction in which a normal human being has to look in order to get the objective constituent under consideration into the middle of his visual field; and that 'this is known to depend *simply* on what is going on in the immediate neighbourhood of his eyes'.[1] In defence of this statement, he cites, for example, the situation in which a mirror reflection may cause a certain place behind the mirror to be occupied ('pervaded') in a certain way, when in fact that place is not so occupied, and another place equidistant in front of the mirror is so occupied.

Now I fail to see how this complication due to mirror reflection (or, for that matter, any of the causal considerations which Dr. Broad cites) justifies the conclusion that the direction, or the position, or the qualitative characteristics of the pervaded region is known to depend *simply* on what is going on in the immediate neighbourhood of the observer's eyes. For it seems undeniable that what is occurring at the mirror, and the position of the mirror —not to mention the position and characteristics of the object which the mirror reflects—are very important factors in determining the position of the region which will appear to the observer to be occupied, and the characteristics which that region will appear to have. It is certainly true, as Dr. Broad says, that the direction of the place of pervasion is determined by the direction in which the light enters the observer's eyes. But it is equally clear that the direction in which the light enters the observer's eyes is determined both by the position of the mirror and the position of the object from which the light is reflected in the first place.

At the conclusion of his argument from complications due to mirrors, however, Dr. Broad rephrases his thesis to read: 'The position of the pervaded region is *immediately* determined by events in or close to the region of projection.'[2] And this provides a clue to the understanding of what otherwise seems to be an absurd claim. For if 'immediately determined' means 'determined chronologically last', then Dr. Broad's assertion becomes a mere truism. Naturally the direction and the characteristics of the light as it enters the observer's eyes are the *final* determinants of the position of the region which will appear to the observer to be occupied, and of the characteristics which that region will appear to him to have.

---

1 *Idem*, p. 165 (italics mine).
2 *Idem*, p. 166 (italics mine).

This raises the point, then, of what, exactly, Dr. Broad means by the phrase 'the independently necessary and sufficient material conditions'. As I understand Dr. Broad's explanation of this phrase,[1] his argument runs something like this. In view of the complications arising from mirror reflection, non-homogeneous media, the finite velocity of light, and the effects of drugs and morbid bodily states, it is necessary in the analysis of perceptual situations to distinguish between the emitting region and its characteristics, on the one hand, and the pervaded region and its apparent characteristics, on the other. Inasmuch as the apparent pervasion of a certain place by a given colour may occur for a certain observer even when this place is actually unoccupied physically, or when it is actually occupied by a totally different set of characteristics, the conditions which are found within the region of projection are themselves *sufficient* for determining the place and characteristics of apparent pervasion. These conditions are the events in the eyes, optic nerves and brain of the observer, and the direction and characteristics of the light as it enters the observer's eyes. Moreover, inasmuch as these conditions are essential to *any* instance of apparent pervasion, regardless of whether or not the pervaded region and the emitting region coincide in place and agree in characteristics, they may be said to be *necessary* conditions for a certain shade of colour to pervade a certain external region from a certain region of projection. This explains the qualifications 'necessary and sufficient'.

Now if the foregoing is correct, then it is clear that the 'microscopic physical events' in the emitting region are *at best* (i.e., in the normal veridical case) only the necessary conditions of these necessary conditions within the region of projection which are the *immediate* determinants of the pervasion of the particular region by the particular shade of colour. And a necessary condition of a necessary condition may be called a 'dependently' necessary condition of that event.[2] Hence, while the events in in the region of projection may be described as *independently* necessary and sufficient, the microscopic physical events in the emitting region are thus only *dependently* necessary.[3]

---

[1] *Idem*, pp. 167 ff.
[2] *Idem*, p. 167.
[3] At this point (*idem*, pp. 169 f.) Dr. Broad also undertakes to explain the importance of the term 'material' in the phrase 'the *independently* necessary and sufficient *material* conditions' 'which occurs in his original answer to the 'causal question'

Turning now to discuss these arguments, admittedly Dr. Broad may legitimately give whatever names he chooses to the distinctions he chooses to make; but if he means not only to tag but also to characterize the distinctions by the names he applies to them— as I think he does—then we are entitled to examine the justification for his characterizations. Now there is a sense in which it may plausibly be argued that a necessary condition of a necessary condition of an event as 'dependently' necessary. It may be dependently necessary, for instance, in the sense that it can bring about the given event only through the mediation of the temporally and geographically more immediate necessary conditions of that event. Thus, if an event r is caused only by conditions q, then q is a necessary condition for r; and if conditions q are in turn caused only by conditions p, then p is a necessary condition for both q and r. It is a necessary condition for r, however, only in virtue of its being a necessary condition for q which operates without further process to cause r. Hence, it may be argued that though p is independently necessary for q, it is *dependently* necessary for r; while q is *independently* necessary for r.

Applying this now to the analysis of perception, the condition p would be the things and events occurring in the emitting region; q would be the conditions within the region of projection; and r would be the fact that there is a certain place which appeared to be pervaded by a certain shade of colour to the observer in the region of projection. Obviously the things and events in the emitting region can cause a certain region to *appear* to be pervaded only through the causal mediation of the temporally and geographically more immediate conditions within the region of projection. In this sense, then, the conditions within the emitting region are *dependently* necessary for the pervasion of the given region, while the conditions within the region of projection are *independently* necessary.

Now so far as the foregoing is concerned, it is not at all clear that there is a point of disagreement between Dr. Broad and the

---

(*supra*). His explanation is that 'we cannot be completely certain that the sensible inherence of such and such a shade of colour in such and such a place from a given region of projection *may* not have psychical as well as physical conditions. Since we cannot get a brain and nervous system like ours working properly without a mind like ours . . .'. Inasmuch as a satisfactory discussion of this point would require a prolonged discussion of the concept 'mind' in Dr. Broad's philosophy, I shall pass up this point as leading us too far afield.

common-sense view. I have already pointed out earlier that inasmuch as 'pervasion' refers to the *appearance* of being occupied, common sense would agree that a necessary condition for a region to be pervaded by a colour is that there be someone to whom the region so appears. Even aside from this consideration, however, I think it is also true that common sense would allow that the conditions in or near the region of projection do play a causally necessary role in the psycho-physical process whereby a certain region appears to a percipient individual to be pervaded by a particular set of characteristics. For it is a matter of common knowledge that we see objects via their emission or reflection of light; and it is platitudinous that the final link in the causal chain involves the sensory apparatus of the percipient individual. Far from denying this fact, common sense explicitly employs it in order to explain those instances of erroneous perception which are due to such factors as colour-blindness, eyestrain, the effects of drugs, non-homogeneous media, etc., within the region of projection. And finally, inasmuch as 'independently' necessary means, as we have seen, *immediately* necessary, it follows that in acknowledging the conditions within the region of projection to be the final necessary causal link for a certain place to be occupied, common sense is also agreeing that—in Dr. Broad's terms—the 'independently' necessary conditions for the pervasion of a certain place by a certain shade of colour are contained in or close to the region of projection. For common sense would not deny that the conditions within the region of projection are temporally and geographically more immediate or final than any preceding conditions in the causal chain outside the region of projection.

6

That the region of projection contains the 'independently necessary' conditions for the pervasion of a certain place by a certain shade of colour is not, then, a point of issue with common sense. The real issue, I believe, centres in Dr. Broad's contention that the conditions within the region of projection are *sufficient* as well as independently necessary. Now in the terminology of logic, it is true, one event is a *sufficient* condition for another event if the latter always occurs when the former does. One event is a *necessary* condition for another event if the former always occurs when the latter does. Thus a given event is both a sufficient and a necessary condition for another only if the second occurs whenever the first does, and does not occur when the first does not. From this, it must be admitted, it follows that the conditions which are to be found in the region of projection are both necessary and sufficient for the sensible pervasion of a given region by a certain shade of colour. For it is true, of course, that in order for anyone to see a coloured object in a given place, the light from the object must reach his eyes, and he must have properly functioning visual apparatus. In this respect, the conditions in the region of projection are necessary; and those in the emitting region are not sufficient. Again, it would seem that whenever the light from the emitting region did reach the eyes of an observer with normally functioning visual apparatus, that observer would certainly see a given place (normally the emitting region) as pervaded. And in this sense the conditions within the region of projection may also be said to be sufficient.

Now I do not think that the common-sense individual would want to take issue with Dr. Broad on the fact that *if* the light from the emitting region *did* reach the eyes of a normal observer, this would be sufficient for the observer to see a given place as occupied. But I think that the following common-sense objection *can* be raised against Dr. Broad's contention that the conditions and events within the region of projection are independently necessary and sufficient for a given region to appear to be occupied. Dr. Broad's assertion seems to suggest that the events in the emitting region are at best causally adventitious to the perception of that region as being occupied. It is as though he were saying that the sole difference between an hallucinatory visual experience in which a certain external place appears to be occupied, and a veridical experience of the same type and content, is that in the latter case there merely *happens* to be an actual object in that place—i.e., there merely *happens* to be an 'emitting region' as well as a 'pervaded region', and the two merely *happen* to coincide. Now the point I want to make is this. Granting that there is a purely technical sense in which the conditions within the region of projection may be held in either case to be 'sufficient' for a given place to appear to be pervaded, there is still a very important difference between an hallucinatory experience and a veridical one. There is a sense in which it is true that the conditions and events within the region of projection are sufficient for the occurrence of an *hallucinatory* visual experience of a given external place as being occupied, but in which it is not likewise true for the occurrence of a *veridical* experience of the same type. The difference between the former sense and this latter one is between the purely logical meaning of the term 'sufficient' and the causal, physical connotation.

Consider, for example, a visual after-image which occurs when we stare intently at a bright light and then look away. In this experience a certain external region may appear to be pervaded by light of a certain colour and shade when in fact no such light physically occupies that region. When this is the case, it is clear that it is the events in the region of projection alone—i.e., the mental and physiological conditions of the observer—which give rise to the visual experience. In this case the events in the region of projection are not only *logically* sufficient for the given external region to appear to be occupied, but they are also *causally* complete and sufficient. But now consider the situation in which under normal conditions we look at a certain place which actually contains a physical object of a given colour and shade, and we see that place as being occupied by that particular object. In this case it may also be said that the logically sufficient conditions for the occurrence of our visual perception of the object are contained within the region of projection. For so long as there is a normal observer in the region of projection and his eyes are stimulated in the proper way, nothing more is needed for him to have the visual experience. But it is perfectly clear in this case, 'in view of what we know of geometrical and physical optics and the physiology of vision'—the causal considerations to which Dr. Broad himself appeals in raising the problem—that the conditions in the region of projection are not the only conditions which are relevant to the perception of this particular object. For this is a veridical perceptual situation; and for a veridical perceptual situation to occur, it is not enough that the observer be in a certain condition in the region of projection. It is essential that there be an actual 'emitting region' containing a physical object, and that light from its surface reach his eyes in the normal fashion—i.e., white light travelling in a straight line through a fairly homogeneous medium. And this clearly takes us outside the region of projection.

THE 'CAUSAL QUESTION'

Dr. Broad is content to limit his account of even the normal perceptual process to the observer in the region of projection and to the light immediately entering the observer's eyes from a given direction. But this is not acceptable to common sense. For it is a matter of common observation and knowledge that the light which enters the observer's eyes in the region of projection has, in normal cases, an external origin. As Dr. Broad himself admits, the physical events within the region of projection, of course, have physical causes outside this region in the emitting region. But if Dr. Broad admits this, in what way, then, is the common-sense notion incorrect? Common sense would not deny that the independently necessary conditions—in the sense that Dr. Broad apparently intends—for a certain region to appear to be occupied by a certain colour are contained in or near the region of projection. Nor is Dr. Broad's argument that *if* the light from the emitting region *does* reach the eyes of the observer with normally functioning visual apparatus, this is sufficient for the observer to see a given place as occupied, in any way contrary to common sense. Common sense would insist, it is true, that such a foreshortened view of the normal perceptual process is artificial; because when we do perceive an object under normal conditions and see it where and as it is, the conditions and events in the region of projection are obviously not the whole story. The light emitted from the object in the emitting region is indispensably necessary to produce and determine *that particular* visual situation, even though the visual situations of dreams or those of the drunkard and his pink rats do have *their* causally sufficient conditions entirely within the region of projection. But Dr. Broad admits, as I have said, that normal perceptual situations do have external physical causes; and though he emphasizes the importance of the conditions and events within the region of projection as having the 'final say', so to speak, as to the location and characteristics of the region which will appear to the observer to be occupied, I cannot believe that he would deny that the actual conditions and events in the emitting region uniquely affect and determine the conditions in the region of projection which are the immediate or independently necessary conditions for this to occur. (For if the object in the emitting region absorbs and reflects light with the wavelength frequency of red, for example, this certainly will determine and affect the conditions and events in the region of projection differently from an object which absorbs and reflects light with the wavelength frequency of, say, green; and if the emitting region is located far to the left of the observer, the region which will appear to him to be occupied will certainly be different from that when the emitting region is nearby and at his right.) And finally, I do not think that Dr. Broad could deny that in the normal case the 'final say' of the 'independently necessary' conditions in the region of projection but acquiesces, so to speak, in the 'earlier say' which the 'dependently necessary' conditions in the emitting region have with respect to the location and characteristics of the region which will appear to the observer to be occupied. For where there are no complications due to mirror-images, non-homogeneous media, astigmatism, or the like, the actual location and characteristics of the emitting region are the only contingent determining factors.[1]

In view of all this, then, I conclude that Dr. Broad has not as yet shown either that the common-sense view cannot be accepted, or even that there is any point of issue between his view and that of common sense, other than a purely verbal one. Dr. Broad tells us that common sense holds that 'the independently necessary and sufficient conditions for the pervasion of a certain region are contained in *that* region'. If this is what the common-sense view comes to in his terms, very well. But then Dr. Broad ought not to employ these terms to mean anything other than what common sense intends. The truth is, however, that the proposition which he understands by these words which he attributes to common sense is not one which common sense either denies or affirms.

---

[1] The qualification 'contingent' is necessary in view of Dr. Broad's statement that the distance of the region which will appear to the observer to be occupied 'is presumably determined by traces left in [his] brain by past visual situations and correlate bodily movements in cases where the vision really was direct and through a homogeneous medium' (*Idem*, p. 166). Inasmuch as Dr. Broad includes such neural considerations in what he calls the 'independently necessary and sufficient conditions' in the region of projection, it is true that even in the normal case the actual location and characteristics of the emitting region are not the *sole* factors determining the location and characteristics of the region which will appear to the observer to be occupied. Nevertheless, in normal cases the actual location and characteristics of the emitting region are the only *unique* or variable determinants in the situation. The traces left in the observer's brain and nervous system and the correlation with bodily movements are established relatively early; and they constitute for all practical purposes a constant set of conditions which he brings to all subsequent sensory experience.

Whether the 'independently necessary and sufficient conditions for the pervasion of a certain region by a certain colour'—in the technical sense in which Dr. Broad uses these terms—are contained in the 'pervaded region' or in the 'region of projection' are philosophers' subtleties which do not enter into the practical concerns of everyday life from which the common-sense notion and language about perception derive. What common sense does hold is simply the empirical fact that—taking these words in their ordinary sense—we do very often perceive the actual location and characteristics of objects, and that when we do, this is causally determined by the actual external physical state of affairs. And this, as Dr. Broad admits, in effect, is true. Thus, it is clear that the disagreement with common sense is not actual.

7

The preceding considerations notwithstanding, I want now to discuss the last item in Dr. Broad's third point of supposed disagreement with common sense. This argument concerning the location of the independently necessary and sufficient conditions for the pervasion of a certain region by a certain colour is that even when there is an emitting region and it coincides with the pervaded region, there is a discrepancy between the date at which the region is pervaded and the date at which the relevant physical events occur in this region. Common sense, Dr. Broad tells us, is in error in that it always assumes that the relevant physical events in the emitting region are contemporary with the pervasion; whereas, due to the finite velocity of light, they are always earlier and may be earlier by thousands of years. Thus, when one looks at a distant star, it might very well be that the star is no longer physically occupying the distant region where it appears to be; in fact, it may actually have disintegrated long before.

With respect to this argument, I want to consider first the extent to which the finite velocity of light justifies the assertion that the independently necessary and sufficient conditions for the pervasion of a certain region are contained in that region. In line with the discussion in the preceding section, I think that the following point is inescapable. The date at which the light (by means of which the observer sees the object) leaves the surface of that object will, regardless of the time required for that light to reach the observer, determine the date at which that object appears to the observer to occupy a certain place. Clearly, if the ray of light which an observer sees at a given moment from a distant star had been emitted from an even more distant star, the date of emission of that particular ray of light would have had to be proportionately earlier. Again, if a certain quiescent star should suddenly flare up into a nova, it is likewise clear that the date at which this appears to an observer on earth is determined by the date at which the relevant physical events occurred. For if they had occurred much later, obviously the star would still appear to be quiescent. These considerations show that while it may be true enough that the events in the region of projection are the *immediately* necessary and sufficient conditions for the observer to see a certain region as pervaded, it is still also true that they are themselves (in non-hallucinatory cases) ultimately determined by the actual events in the emitting region. No matter what happens to the light from the distant star during its journey to earth and into the region of projection, and no matter how long this journey may take, the final apparent characteristics of the light and the date at which the distant region will appear to be occupied by this particular star are as much the resultant of the original events in the emitting region as of the subsequent events in the region of projection. The psycho-physical process of perception is a continuous one and cannot plausibly be separated.

I want to consider next Dr. Broad's assertion that common sense always assumes that the relevant physical events in the emitting region are contemporary with the pervasion of this region, and that hence common sense is always wrong about the date of the former. Now it is true that visual perception of objects occurs via the medium of light rays reflected or emitted from objects. And inasmuch as sight occurs 'at a distance', so to speak, and inasmuch as the velocity of light is measurably finite, it would seem on first consideration that we always see objects as they *were* rather than as they *are*. This argument seems especially compelling when we consider the case of seeing a distant star. Because of the great distance of the stars from the earth, it is, of course, possible that some of the stars which now appear to us to occupy certain regions in the heavens may long ago have left those particular regions, and may even have disintegrated and ceased to exist as stars. In such cases, it must be admitted, the date at which it appears that a star is at a given place may not accord with the date at which it actually is or was at this place. And it would seem that the perception of nearby objects differs from the perception of distant stars only in degree, and that there must inevitably be some lag between the date at which the light that stimulates our eyes leaves the surface of the object, and the date at which it reaches our eyes. Thus, Dr. Broad would seem here to be raising a valid objection to the common-sense belief about perception.

But now I do not think that this argument, which seems so plausible on first consideration, is really tenable. To begin with, let us consider the assertion that common sense always assumes that the 'relevant physical events' in the 'emitting region' are contemporary with the pervasion of this region. So far as I can make out, what Dr. Broad must mean by the 'relevant physical events' is the reflection or emission of the light rays from the surface of an object. Now if he does mean this, then I think he is clearly mistaken in what he is attributing to common sense. For, were the average common-sense individual to know anything about the physics of visual perception, I think it is highly unlikely that he would hold so absurd a notion as that the light from the surface of an object could traverse a finite distance without consuming any time in the journey. The truth is that the common-sense notion about perception has nothing to do with light rays leaving the surface of objects. What common-sense does hold, rather, is that the objects which we see are where they appear to be at the time we see them. Now we have seen that in the case of distant stars it may be that the star which appears to be in a certain region of the heavens may no longer be there. And I think it must be granted that very likely most common-sense individuals are not aware of this fact. Hence it would seem that many common-sense observers *may* be mistaken in what they implicitly believe about the simultaneity of some visual situations involving distant stars.

It is quite another matter, however, when we ask whether common sense is mistaken in what it believes about *ordinary* perceptual situations, involving relatively nearby objects. Here I think it can be shown that what common sense holds about the simultaneous presence of the object at the place at the place where it is seen is not at all untenable in the sense in which common sense holds this. Now again it must be borne in mind that the common-sense individual normally has no occasion either to affirm or to deny the simultaneous presence of an object which he sees. And so it is very unlikely that he has any clearly formulated opinion about this question. Nevertheless, I think it must be granted that there is in some respect an element of simultaneity implicitly involved in the common-sense notion of perception. The common-sense observer does implicitly hold, I believe, that the objects which he sees under normal circumstances are actually 'there' at the time he sees them, and that, allowing for minor inaccuracies of discrimination, they actually have the characteristics at that time which they appear to him to have. But now, if this proposition is to be an accurate rendering of what common sense does actually assume implicitly about perception, and not merely a straw man to serve the purposes of Dr. Broad's argument, then the phrase 'at the time he sees them' must be understood not in the sense of a theoretical 'instant', but rather as a roughly-defined experienceable period of duration, of sufficient length for the observer to discern his error if he is mistaken. For I think that whatever beliefs common sense does hold about perception are only such as have practical significance for concrete experience. If we bear this in mind, then I think it can be shown that common sense is quite correct in what it means to hold.

Suppose we are looking at a static nearby object, steadily, for all of a given minute. Now the speed of light, it will be recalled, is approximately 186,000 miles per second; and this means that for any object within a range of one mile from us, the time required for the light from its surface to reach our eyes is $1/186,000$th of second, or less. Thus, it is clear that if we were to judge at any given time after $1/186,000$th of the first second of the given minute has elapsed, that we are seeing the object *as it is during that given minute*, we would be correct. For, the time it takes for the light rays to reach our eyes notwithstanding, the fact remains that the object is revealed to us as it is at some time during the given minute. But now it is also clear, in view of the enormous speed of light, that we could correctly make this judgment even if the period specified were reduced to a single second. It would still be true, so long as it was made after the first $1/186,000$th part of that second had elapsed, that we were seeing the object as it was at that time—i.e., at some time during the given second. If the judgment were made *before* the first 1/186,000th part of *this* second had elapsed, moreover, it would still be true, of course, for a slightly earlier period of one second which overlapped it. But, then, it is obvious that it would also be true for *any* period of time that the common-sense individual would have in mind. For any such period would at least be long enough for the observer to *have* the visual experience with respect to which he entertains the implicit belief that the object he sees is 'there' at the time he sees it. And this would certainly exceed (in the case of relatively nearby objects) the infinitesimal time lag due to the finite velocity of light.

To sum up the point, then, the period of time intended in the common-sense belief that the objects we see are 'there' when and as we see them, is not a theoretical instant, but is rather an appreciable duration. The time required for the light to reach our eyes from nearby objects is so minute as to defy even careful scientific measurement, let alone unaided perceptual discrimination; and hence it is well within the roughly defined limits intended in the common-sense belief. It is so short, in fact, in the vast majority of cases, that even before we are able to entertain any doubts about the simultaneity of the object we are seeing with our visual experience of it, succeeding light rays at once confirm its continuous unchanging presence. In no case of direct visual perception except that of seeing stellar bodies, or, perhaps, rapidly moving objects, does the finite velocity of light raise the possibility that we are 'seeing something' which is no longer 'there' at the time we see it. And thus it is clear that Dr. Broad's reference to the finite velocity of light does not really challenge this belief insofar as ordinary cases of perception are concerned, so long as the belief is understood in the sense in which common sense holds it.

We have seen, then, in examining the three points on which Dr. Broad alleges common sense to be in error, that none of the causal considerations which he cites are fatal to the common-sense notion of perception. Though mirror-images, jaundice, and the finite velocity of light may sometimes complicate perceptual situations, there is nothing about such abnormal cases which contradicts common-sense beliefs, or which cannot be adequately explained in common-sense terms. And when the perceptual situation is normal, as Dr. Broad himself recognizes, there is not even *prima facie* reason to suppose that the common-sense view cannot be maintained. The net result of the arguments in this chapter and the preceding one has been to show that the common-sense notions about perception and the characteristics of physical objects are perfectly correct in the sense in which they are held and in which they must be understood.

CHAPTER VI

THE SENSUM THEORY

I N Chapter IV we saw that the problem which Dr. Broad feels
concerning the different appearances which an object may
present from different perspectives and under different
conditions leads him to conclude that 'we are tied down to three
alternatives, each almost as distasteful to common sense as the
others'. Thus far I have considered two of these three alternative
solutions which Dr. Broad describes: the Multiple Inherence
Theory and the Multiple Relation Theory of Appearing. In this
chapter I want to consider the third, which Dr. Broad himself
favours: the Sensum Theory.

Like the two we have already considered, the solution which
the Sensum Theory provides similarly turns out upon careful
examination to be merely verbal in character. But the consideration of this 'theory' is of special importance for the argument of
the essay. For as I shall try to show, the Sensum Theory is not
merely, like the others, gratuitous, but is actually assumed by
Dr. Broad, in its essential aspects, from the outset, and is thus the
source of the very pseudo-problem the 'alternative theories' are
supposed to solve.

I

As we saw, Dr. Broad divides the three alternatives into two
major types. One type tries to keep the common-sense view that
the objective constituents of some visual situations are literally
spatio-temporal parts of the particular physical objects which
we are said to be 'seeing'; the other abandons this claim. The
theories which we have already considered are both of the first

type. The Multiple Inherence Theory, we have seen, replies to the problem of the apparent inconsistency of the different appearances of an object with the postulation that 'the physical object can be both constant and variable in its spatial characteristics within the same stretch of time'. This 'distasteful alternative', as I have shown, is Dr. Broad's rendering of the notion that sensible characteristics such as shape, size and colour ought to be regarded—in view of their apparent variability with position and conditions—not as 'intrinsic' properties of objects, but rather as characteristics the specification of which should involve an essential reference to a 'region of projection' or observer-at-a-certain-place-of-observation.

The Multiple Relation Theory of Appearing, on the other hand, meets the alleged problem by holding that the objective constituents of the supposedly incompatible perceptual situations 'can have qualities which are different from and inconsistent with those which they seem on careful inspection to have'. And this 'distasteful alternative', as we saw, turns out, on careful inspection, to be nothing more than the familiar common-sense view that a statement of the form: 'This *looks* blue from here' (asserted of a given object seen under non-ideal conditions), is not necessarily incompatible with a statement of the form: 'This *is really* green', asserted of the same object.

The third alternative which Dr. Broad presents is of the second type. This, the Sensum Theory, abandons the common-sense view that the objective constituents of visual situations can be literally spatio-temporal parts of external objects, and assumes that they are always objects in their own right, 'particular existents of a peculiar kind'. Unlike the Multiple Inherence Theory, the Sensum Theory does not maintain that the different appearances which a round penny, for example, presents under different conditions and from different perspectives, all actually 'inhere' in one particular object, from different regions of projection. And unlike the Multiple Relation Theory, which in effect denies 'that we are aware of *anything* that *really is* elliptical when we have the experience which we express by saying that the penny looks elliptical to us', and which 'assumes a unique and unanalysable multiple relation of "appearing"', the Sensum Theory involves 'a peculiar kind of object—an "appearance"'; and it holds that 'such objects actually *do have* the characteristics which the physical object seems to have'.[1]

The Sensum Theory, Dr. Broad explains,[2] allows that the objective constituents of perceptual situations really do have all those positive characteristics which they seem on careful inspection to have. And it allows that these characteristics inhere in these objective constituents 'in the straightforward dyadic way in which common sense supposes them to do'. No doubt, says Dr. Broad, the objective constituents 'are really extended; they really last for so long; they really have certain shapes, sizes, colours, etc.; and some at least of them stand in spatial and temporal relations to each other'. At this point, however, the Sensum Theory departs from common sense. For on this theory, the objective constituents 'are not, in any plain straightforward sense, in the one Physical Space in which physical objects are supposed to be; and between pairs of them which are connected with different observers there are no simple and straightforward spatial or temporal relations'. Thus, the Sensum Theory cannot admit that when a man says that he is 'seeing and feeling the same object', there is in general a common objective constituent to his visual and his tactual situations, Dr. Broad tells us. Nor can it admit that the visual situations of a number of observers who say that they are 'seeing the same object' contain a common objective constituent. And finally, it cannot admit that, when we say that we are 'seeing a certain physical object', the objective constituent of our visual situation is in general a spatio-temporal part of the physical object which we say that we are 'seeing'.

Dr. Broad writes:

The objective constituents of perceptual situations are, on this view, particular existents of a peculiar kind; they are not physical, as we have seen; and there is no reason to suppose that they are either states of mind or existentially mind-dependent. In having spatial characteristics, colours, etc., they resemble physical objects, as ordinarily conceived; but in their privacy and their dependence on the body, if

---

[1] *Scientific Thought*, p. 237. The preceding chapters of this essay have been concerned with Dr. Broad's argument mainly as it occurs in Ch. IV ('Sense-Perception and Matter') of *The Mind and Its Place in Nature* (1925). In this chapter I refer also to his somewhat more detailed and expanded statement of his views in Chs. VII and VIII ('Matter and Its Appearances', and 'The Theory of Sensa, and the Critical Scientific Theory') of *Scientific Thought* (1923).

[2] *The Mind and Its Place in Nature*, pp. 181 ff.

not the mind, of the observer they are more like mental states. I give the name of 'sensa' to the objective constituents of perceptual situations, on the supposition that they are *not* literally parts of the physical object which we are supposed to be 'perceiving', and that they *are* transitory particulars of the peculiar kind which I have just been describing. And I call the theory which assumes the existence of such particulars 'The Sensum Theory'.[1]

Thus, instead of trying either to preserve the view that the objective constituents of visual situations are literally parts of external physical objects, or to reconcile the different appearances of what is commonly held to be a single object (as do the former two theories which we have considered—neither of which accords very well with common sense, anyway, Dr. Broad believes), the Sensum Theory abandons both attempts and advises common sense 'to follow the example of Judas Iscariot, and "go out and hang itself"'.[2] The solution which it proposes instead is, in effect, to *change the subject*. The different appearances which a circular penny, for example, present to a number of different observers, or to a single observer from different places, are no longer held to constitute a common objective constituent which is literally a part of that one physical object which the single observer or the several observers are said, on the common-sense view, to be seeing. Rather, the statement that the round penny (seen from an oblique perspective) looks to me elliptical is analysed, on the Sensum Theory, into 'a statement which involves the actual existence of an elliptical object, which stands in a certain cognitive relation to me on the one hand, and in another relation, yet to be determined, to the round penny'.[3] Now on the previous two theories, Dr. Broad observes, the relation of the objective constituent to the physical object was relatively direct and simple; in favourable cases the objective constituent was held to be quite literally a spatio-temporal part of the perceived object. But on the Sensum Theory, which does not admit this, the relation is more complicated and less direct than

---

[1] *Idem*, pp. 181 f. Writing in 1923, Dr. Broad says: 'This type of theory, though it has been much mixed up with irrelevant matter, and has never been clearly stated and worked out till our own day, is of respectable antiquity. The doctrine of "representative ideas" is the traditional and highly muddled form of it. It lies at the basis of such works as Russell's *Lowell Lectures on the External World*.' (*Scientific Thought*, p. 238.)

[2] *The Mind and Its Place in Nature*, p. 186.   [3] *Scientific Thought*, pp. 237 f.

THE SENSUM THEORY

common sense believes. On the Sensum Theory, the analysis of the proposition: 'The physical object which I am now perceiving appears to have the determinate characteristics c', Dr. Broad tells us, would yield the following meaning:

> There is a certain sensum s which is the objective constituent of this perceptual situation. This actually has the characteristic c which I can detect in it by inspection, and it has this characteristic in a straightforward dyadic way. And there is a certain physical object o, to which this sensum has a certain relation R which it has to no other physical object. In virtue of this relation the sensum s is said to be 'an appearance of' the physical object o.[1]

On this theory, then, Dr. Broad tells us, when we say that several people perceive the same physical object o and the same part of it, we must mean that their several perceptual situations contain as objective constituents the sensa $s_1, s_2, \ldots$ etc., and that all of them are appearances of the same physical object o. These analyses, Dr. Broad points out, contain an unanalysed factor, the relation R of 'being an appearance of'. This relation is not that of spatio-temporal part to spatio-temporal whole. Many different sensa can be appearances of one physical object, and even of precisely the same part of this object; but, he further explains, one sensum cannot, in this sense, be an appearance of several physical objects. 'There is a certain physical object and a certain part of it which can be called "*the* part of *the* physical object which has this sensum as an appearance".'[2]

At this point, according to Dr. Broad, the Sensum Theory can take one of two courses with respect to the relation of objective constituents or sensa to 'physical objects'. It may abandon the common-sense notion of physical objects and hold 'with Berkeley that what are manifested by sensa are volitions in God's mind; or with Leibniz that what are manifested by sensa are collections of minds; or with Russell that the sensa which are the objective constituents of perceptual situations are a small selection out of certain larger groups of interrelated sensa, and that these groups are the only physical objects that there are'.[3] The second course would be to try to keep as close to the common-sense notion of physical objects as possible. The latter course, says Dr. Broad, leads to the 'Critical Scientific Theory', which is the

---

[1] *The Mind and Its Place in Nature*, p. 182.
[2] *Idem*, p. 183. [3] *Ibid.*

THE SENSUM THEORY

'tacit assumption of natural scientists, purged of its inconsistencies, and stated in terms of the Sensum Theory'; but he does not believe that this is an ultimately satisfactory position.[1]

Dr. Broad, as I have said, favours the Sensum Theory over the two theories which we have already considered as alternatives to the common-sense view. Writing in 1923 of the Multiple Relation Theory of Appearing, Dr. Broad says: 'Theories of this type have been suggested lately by Professor Dawes Hicks and by Dr. G. E. Moore. So far, they have not been worked out in any great detail, but they undoubtedly deserve careful attention.'[2] These remarks notwithstanding, however, there can be no doubt that Dr. Broad's predilection is all for the Sensum or 'Object' type theory, rather than for the Multiple Relation Theory which, as we have seen, is hardly more than a formal statement of the common-sense view. Though he tells us that he does not regard the argument for the Sensum Theory as absolutely conclusive, 'because I am inclined to think that the Multiple Relation Theory can explain these facts also', nevertheless the treatment of perception in *Scientific Thought*, at least, is entirely in terms of the notion of sensa; and he pleads that it must at least be admitted that the sensum theory is 'highly plausible'.[3]

In *The Mind and Its Place in Nature*, on the other hand, where, as we have seen, he does give some attention to the Multiple Relation Theory and to the Multiple Inherence Theory, before presenting the Sensum Theory, Dr. Broad concludes, following a consideration of the three alternatives, that:

> The upshot of this discussion seems to me to be that, on the whole, there are no greater objections to the Sensum Theory than to the other theories, and that the other theories have no positive advantages over the Sensum Theory when carefully considered. And, as the Sensum Theory does not require to assume Absolute Space-time as a pre-existing matrix, while the other theories apparently do, the balance of advantage seems to be slightly on the side of the Sensum Theory.[4]

Now I have already shown that the fact that an object presents different appearances under different conditions and from different perspectives does not constitute any real problem for the common-sense view of perception; and that, quite on the contrary, there are perfectly adequate explanations for such

---

[1] Cf. *Scientific Thought*, p. 282   [2] *Idem*, p. 237
[3] *Idem*, p. 240.   [4] P. 195.

phenomena in common-sense terms which do not require the questionable services of either the Multiple Inherence Theory or the Multiple Relation Theory of Appearing. Consequently there would be little point in following Dr. Broad in the intricacies of whether or not these theories do 'require to assume Absolute Space-Time as a pre-existing matrix', whatever this might mean. However, I do want to try to make clear just why Dr. Broad finds so bizarre and complicated a notion as the Sensum Theory, which requires us to assume the existence of such peculiar non-physical, non-mental 'entities' as sensa, *at all* plausible, let alone more plausible than the familiar and pragmatically successful common-sense view. And I think that the answer to this question lies not in such technical matters as whether or not the alternative theories involve 'Absolute Space-Time as a pre-existing matrix', but rather in the more fundamental matter of Dr. Broad's analysis of perception, as I shall try to show presently.

2

The Multiple Relation Theory and the common-sense view, as I have already indicated, have one important thing in common which distinguishes them from the Sensum Theory and from the Multiple Inherence Theory. This is that they in effect deny that when a round penny, for example, *appears* to us to be elliptical (in the sense in which this might be said when the penny is viewed from an oblique perspective), there is any*thing* that 'really is' elliptical which we can properly be said to be seeing. Now in support of the Sensum Theory, Dr. Broad offers three examples to show that it is highly plausible to take the view that in all such cases there *really is* something of which we are aware that *really has* the characteristics which the physical object *seems to have*: viz., a 'sensum'. The three examples are designed to make clear the distinction between sensa and physical objects. Let us examine them briefly.

Dr. Broad's first example is concerned with the already familiar case of the elliptical appearance which a round penny presents when seen from the side:

When I look at a penny from the side I am certainly aware of some-*thing*; and it is certainly plausible to hold that this something is elliptical in the same plain sense in which a suitably bent piece of wire, looked at from straight above, is elliptical. If, in fact, nothing elliptical is before my mind, it is very hard to understand why the penny should seem *elliptical* rather than of any other shape.[1]

The second example which Dr. Broad presents involves the case of looking at a straight stick which is half in water and half in air. In such cases, Dr. Broad points out, we say that the stick looks bent. However, he observes:

... we certainly do not mean by this that we mistakenly judge it to be bent; we generally make no such mistake. We are aware of an object which is very much like what we should be aware of if we were looking at a stick with a physical kink in it, immersed wholly in air. The most obvious analysis of the facts is that, when we judge that a straight stick *looks* bent, we are aware of an object which really *is* bent, and which is related in a peculiarly intimate way to the physically straight stick. The relation cannot be that of identity; since the same thing cannot at once be bent and straight in the same sense of these words. If there be *nothing* with a kink in it before our minds at the moment, why should we think then of kinks at all, as we do when we say that the stick looks bent? No doubt we can quite well mistakenly *believe* a property to be present which is really absent, when we are dealing with something which is only known to us indirectly, like Julius Caesar or the North Pole. But in our example we are dealing with a concrete visible object which is bodily present to our senses; and it is very hard to understand how we could seem to ourselves to *see* the property of bentness exhibited in a concrete instance, if in fact *nothing* was present to our minds that possessed that property.[2]

Finally, Dr. Broad's third example has to do with the assertion which he says scientists often make, that physical objects are not 'really' red or hot. 'We are not at present concerned with the truth or falsehood of this strange opinion,' Dr. Broad tells us, 'but only with its application to our present problem.'

When a scientist looks at a penny stamp or burns his mouth with a potato he has exactly the same sort of experience as men of baser clay, who know nothing of the scientific theories of light and heat. The visual experience seems to be adequately described by saying that each of them is aware of a red patch of approximately square shape. If such patches be not in fact red, and if people be not in fact aware of such patches, where could the notion of red or of any other

[1] *Scientific Thought*, p. 240.
[2] *Idem*, p. 241.

colour have come from? The scientific theory of colour would have nothing to explain, unless people really are aware of patches under various circumstances which really do have different colours. . . . Thus we seem forced to the view that there are at least hot and coloured sensa; and, if we accept the scientific view that physical objects are neither hot nor coloured, it will follow that sensa cannot be identified with physical objects.[1]

I want now to comment briefly on each of these examples. Concerning the first, I do not think that anything more is required to be said than I have already said in the discussion of the similar argument in Chapter IV. As Dr. Broad himself concedes, he is inclined to think that the Multiple Relation Theory can explain these facts also. And I have shown that, stripped of its formal phraseology, the Multiple Relation Theory is nothing but the common-sense view.

Turning next to the second example, I think this too may be disposed of fairly quickly. What Dr. Broad is concerned with is how it is possible that in looking at a straight stick immersed partly in air and partly in water, we should see it as having a kink in it. The stick has no kink in it *actually*, yet we do see *something* which has a kink in it. Now the scientific explanation of this phenomenon is, of course, a matter of common knowledge. It is to be found in physical optics. We know that in such a situation we should be seeing the stick through two different media; and we know that the refractive powers of these two media, air and water, differ, water being more dense than air. In passing from the denser medium to the less dense, the light which is reflected to our eyes from that part of the stick which is immersed in the water is bent away from the perpendicular; while the light which is reflected from that part of the stick not immersed in the water does not pass from one medium into another, and hence is not similarly refracted. Thus the stick appears to be bent at the point at which it is immersed in water.

To this explanation, however, Dr. Broad would likely reply as he does to the explanation involving the facts about perspective and the physics of light (Chapter IV, Sec. 7). He would probably say: 'It is quite true that we can *predict what particular appearance* an object will present to an observer when we know the shape of the object and the refractive indices of the media through which

[1] *Idem*, p. 242.

it is observed. But all we know in that case is what shape to expect through given media. Our question is as to the compatibility of these changing appearances of shape, however they may be correlated with other facts in the world, with the supposed constancy and straightness of the physical object.'[1] But if he does say this, I must also reply as I did then. I am at a loss to understand what he is asking. For surely these facts about the different refractive indices of different media *do* explain the phenomenon of the bent appearance of the stick. And there is hence no need to postulate the existence of sensa. Dr. Broad might as well say that the fact that a thumb was partly obscured by a piece of string across it would be sufficient reason to say that what we would be seeing if we looked at it was not to be identified with the thumb, or any part of it, because what we would see is something with a piece of string across it, whereas the common-sense notion of a thumb doesn't involve its having a piece of string across it. Of course, our notion of straight sticks doesn't involve their being seen partly immersed in water. Yet, clearly it is correct to say in the first case that what we see is the thumb partly obscured by the piece of string; and, by the same token, that in the second case it is the stick partly obscured by water (only in this case in the way that such an imperfectly transparent medium obscures—i.e., with a refractive effect).

Thus, we *know* why we should 'think of kinks' even though the stick itself is not kinked. Owing to refraction, the light which is reflected from the stick actually forms a bent pattern which impinges upon the retina of our eye, and which would affect a photographic film in the same pattern. We don't have to suppose that there is a *thing* which is kinked, unless we want to speak of the pattern of reflected light rays as a *thing*. If we do, however, we had better be careful to bear in mind just what sort of a 'thing' it is.

Finally, with respect to the third example, I cannot agree with Dr. Broad that the truth or falsehood of this strange opinion which he attributes to scientists is not relevant to the problem at issue. For if this notion is mistaken, as I think it very obviously is, then Dr. Broad has neither shown by this example that there are such things as sensa, nor, *a fortiori*, that the objective constituents of visual situations cannot be identified with physical objects.

That the strange opinion which he attributes to scientists is

[1] Cf. *idem*, pp. 235 f.

hopelessly muddled (as Dr. Broad in fact seems to recognize), there can be no doubt. Whatever it is that those scientists whom Dr. Broad has in mind want to say, they cannot correctly say that physical objects are never red or hot—if these words are to be understood in their literal ordinary senses. Of course, physicists as such are not concerned with the sense qualities of objects. They have no need in their procedures for qualitative terms like 'hot' or 'red'. They are concerned rather with giving quantitative equivalents for such terms in the systematization of physical phenomena. But it no more follows from the fact that they can do this, nor from the fact that they can dispense with such qualitative observations and terms, that objects aren't ever 'really' red or hot, than it follows from the fact that tables and chairs can theoretically be described in terms of molecules and atoms, that there aren't 'really' such things as tables and chairs.[1] It would be very strange indeed if merely by giving a causal analysis of the process by which we perceive the sensible qualitative characteristics of objects, the scientist could cause those characteristics to disappear!

I conclude, then, that Dr. Broad has failed, at least so far as the argument of these three examples is concerned, to demonstrate either that there are sensa or that the objective constituents of visual situations cannot in general be identified with external physical objects. He has not, in fact, succeeded in making clear at all what he means by a sensum. However, from his statement that on this theory 'all that I ever come to know about physical objects and their qualities seems to be based upon the qualities of the sensa that I become aware of in sense-perception',[2] it would seem that he is espousing what might suggestively be called a 'television' theory of perception. He distinguishes between the physical object which we should ordinarily say was present before our eyes (in the analogy: before the lens of the television camera), and what is 'before our minds' (the televised image produced on the screen). The television audience does not see the original object, but only an image of it. Similarly, Dr. Broad holds that we do not see the object directly, but only through the medium of sensa, as though the latter were a peculiar kind of 'image', neither physical nor mental, of parts of the surfaces

1 Cf. S. Stebbing, *Philosophy and the Physicists*.
2 *Scientific Thought*, p. 241.

of physical objects. Now, of course, Dr. Broad does not concede that sensa necessarily reveal external physical objects as these are ordinarily conceived. For, as we have seen, he suggests that physical objects might be regarded, as Bertrand Russell does, or once did, regard them, as merely 'logical constructs', small selections out of 'certain larger groups of interrelated sensa', these groups being the only physical objects that there are. But I think that the analogy holds, at least in the following respect. In the case of television, perception of the original object is *mediated* by the technical process involving the television camera, electronic transmission, and the receiving and reproducing apparatus. Hence, if there is a discrepancy between the resultant image and the original object, this discrepancy can be explained as due to the faultiness of the reproduction. The error is explicable because of the mediation. If perception were non-mediated, or *direct*, the presence of error would be inexplicable.

I have shown, however, that the examples that Dr. Broad cites do not require us to adopt this device. There is no need for, nor is there any unambiguous evidence to support, the view that our perception of physical objects is mediated by sensa. Instead of adopting an object type of mediation, we may simply recognize that our perception is a process involving the reflection of light; and this is sufficient to account adequately for all those peculiar phenomena of perception to which Dr. Broad calls our attention. We have thus uprooted Dr. Broad's fundamental argument for the Sensum Theory by explaining in familiar common-sense terms the supposed occurrence of 'discrepancy' in our perception of physical objects. There is nothing for the Sensum Theory to explain that can't be adequately handled by scientific investigation in a way wholly compatible with common sense; and hence the theory is gratuitous.

3

The critical discussion thus far has been directed toward showing the speciousness of the 'logical problem' which the Sensum Theory is designed to solve. I propose now to turn attention to the character of the solution which the theory provides. And I want to begin by showing a certain paradox which confronts Dr. Broad's attempt to meet the objection that we are not as a rule aware of sensa and their properties, and that this constitutes good reason for doubting that sensa, at least ordinarily, mediate our perception of physical objects.

It is a fact, Dr. Broad says, that it often needs a good deal of persuasion to make a man believe that, when he looks at a penny from the side, it seems elliptical to him.[1] And, accordingly, it is argued that we have no right to believe that such a man is directly sensing an object which is, in fact, elliptical.

Now we must distinguish, according to Dr. Broad, between failing to notice what is present in an object, and 'noticing' what is not present in an object. In the case of the penny, it is only when we are looking at a penny almost normally that any doubt is felt of the ellipticity of the sensum, he observes; and in that case the sensum is, in fact, very nearly round. But it is no objection to the Sensum Theory, we are told, that a sensum which is not quite round should be thought to be exactly round; though it would be an objection if an exactly round sensum seemed to be elliptical. The reason is that an ellipse, with its variable curvature, is a more 'differentiated' figure than a circle, with its uniform curvature. For instance, he says, a man might think on inspecting one of his sensa, that it was exactly round and uniformly red, and be mistaken. But 'exactly round' means 'with no variation of curvature'; and 'uniformly red' means 'with no variation of shade from one part to another'. Now universal judgments like these, Dr. Broad says, can never be guaranteed by mere inspection; and so, in such cases, the man is not 'seeing properties which are not there' in the sense in which he would be doing so if a round sensum appeared to him to be elliptical. There is no difficulty in the fact that we overlook minute differentiations that are really present in our sensa, he says; difficulties would arise only if we seemed to notice distinctions that are not really present, for

[1] *Scientific Thought*, p. 246. This persuasion, Dr. Broad here tells us, is unfortunately all too often brought about by 'some absurd and irrelevant argument that the area of his retina affected by the light from the penny is an oblique projection of a circle, and is therefore an ellipse'. But only 'direct inspection' is relevant evidence, Dr. Broad insists. It seems strange that Dr. Broad should not avail himself of what would seem to be an extremely strong argument, until we realize that if this causal explanation is allowed, it obviates the necessity for the Sensum Theory; for in the very argument itself lies the scientific explanation for the phenomenon out of which Dr. Broad seems determined to generate a problem! (For further comment on Dr. Broad's inconsistency with respect to the appeal to causal considerations, see *supra*, Ch. IV, Sec. 7, and Ch. V, Sec. 1, esp. ftn. 1.)

then the same difficulties would break out in the Sensum Theory that it was put forward to solve.[1]

Thus, according to Dr. Broad, while sensa cannot appear to have properties which they do not really have, they may have more properties than we do or can notice in them. And there is no difficulty whatever, he says, in supposing that two sensa may really differ in quality when we think that they are exactly alike.[2]

Now I think that there is a very central difficulty involved in this notion, which I want to try to show. Dr. Broad says that we must distinguish between failing to notice what is present in an object and 'noticing' what is not present in an object. I want to consider the notion of 'failing to notice what is present in an object'.

Suppose we were permitted to view an intricately patterned diagram for a brief span of time, after which it was withdrawn from our view. Under such conditions, it is, of course, extremely likely that we should fail to notice some of its qualities. Perhaps it was composed mostly of rectangles, with a few very small curved figures interspersed; and on being presented with it, we failed to notice the curved figures among the predominating rectangular ones. Or, it might be a colour kaleidoscope, consisting mostly of, say, reds, greens, and browns, with one or two orange-coloured bits strewn about the visible field. In that case, too, it might very likely happen that we should fail to notice the orange colour amidst the preponderance of red, green, and brown, even though the orange-coloured bits were visible in the sense that they were not physically obscured.

Now the question I want to raise is this. What does it mean to say that we failed to notice a quality that was *actually present*? But this question is inextricably bound up with the further question of what this comes to, ultimately: How could we tell that we had failed to notice a quality that was actually present? In other words, what is the difference—aside from the obvious difference in the words employed—between the situation represented by the phrase 'failed to notice a quality actually present', and that represented by the phrase '*did not* fail to notice a quality actually present'? The answer to this question, it seems to me, must be something to the effect that on further inspection of *the same object*, we notice what we did not previously notice; or

---

[1] *Idem*, pp. 244 ff.   [2] *Idem*, p. 244.

else, that others inspecting *the same object* report it more fully than we do. It follows, then, that if it is to signify a meaningful possibility to say that we might fail to notice a quality that was actually present in a given thing or situation, that thing or situation must be capable of repeated inspection in some way.

If the thing in question is a physical object, of course, in the ordinary sense in which this term is understood, this requirement presents no difficulty. We may inspect the same object at different times and in different ways; and others may simultaneously or subsequently inspect it too. But now let us consider this matter with respect to sensa. Sensa, as Dr. Broad tells us, 'do seem to be private to each observer. . . . It is at least doubtful whether two people, who say that they are perceiving the same object, are ever sensing the same sensum or even two precisely similar sensa.'[1] And in the same place he goes on to explain: 'Since no two men's bodies can be in precisely the same place at precisely the same time, it is not surprising that the sensa of the two men should differ. And, since the internal states and the minute structures of no two living bodies are exactly alike, it is still less surprising.'

From the preceding, then, it would seem that it cannot be on the basis of the testimony of others that one could determine that one of his sensa had had qualities which he had failed to notice. The only possibility left, then, is that he discover this through subsequent or else previous inspection. This, however, raises the very crucial question of whether or not it is possible to examine precisely the same sensum on two different occasions, and, what is more important, whether or not it is possible to *know* that one was examining precisely the same sensum. Now it must be admitted that I have nowhere been able to find in Dr. Broad's writings an explicit statement to the effect that a single individual *cannot* experience one and the same sensum at two different times. Nor is there any clear statement to be found concerning the temporal period during which one can properly be said to be 'seeing the same sensum'. There is, however, some evidence to show that, on Dr. Broad's view, temporally distinct perceptions reveal numerically different sensa. Inasmuch as he seems to know—surprisingly, it may be noted, in view of the doubts which would seem to be cast on all such knowledge by the Sensum Theory—that the internal states and the minute structures of

[1] *Idem*, p. 259.

no two living bodies are exactly alike, and that this as well as differences in place and time are relevant to the characteristics which one's sensa will appear to have, it would seem to follow that the fact that even one and the same individual (whatever that would mean on this theory) is in a different state, from one moment to another, precludes the possibility of his seeing precisely the same sensum from moment to moment, or even ever again. And in any case, there would be no way, even theoretically, of deciding that a given sensum was the same as that which one had previously seen. (Even if it seemed to the individual that his bodily state, etc., had not changed relevantly from one moment to the next while he thought he was inspecting the same sensum, it may be pointed out, this would not be conclusive; for on Dr. Broad's own argument, there is no difficulty in supposing that the individual may have *failed to notice* a subtle but relevant change in his bodily state.)

Dr. Broad, as a matter of fact, seems to recognize the difficulty to which I am pointing; but his reply would indicate that he has not fully appreciated its fatal consequences. The passage to which I refer occurs in his discussion of the possibility of inspecting a 'sense field'.[1] As anyone who has tried to discover the apparent qualities of his visual or auditory sensa, as distinct from trying to discover the physical qualities of external objects, knows, he writes, it is utterly different to inspect a sensum and to perceive with it. This raises the question whether we can do both with respect to the same sensum. Dr. Broad admits that it is doubtful whether we can; and he says that when we are tempted to think that we do so, we are really alternating quickly to and fro between 'perceiving with' and 'inspecting'. And this raises the problem that if what one inspects be probably never numerically the same as what one has perceived with, what right does one have to believe that the objective constituent of the past perceptual situation *had* (or *would have* seemed to have) those characteristics which the objective constituent of the present inspective situation *does* now seem to have?

In reply to this question, Dr. Broad admits that no conclusive reason can be given for this belief. However, he explains this as being due to the fact that it involves a memory judgment; and the correctness of memory in general, he tells us, cannot be

[1] *The Mind and Its Place in Nature*, pp. 297 ff.

proved by argument. It *may* be, he says, that the characteristics which the objective constituent of an inspective situation seem to have are always different from those which the objective constituent of the immediately previous perceptual situation had or seemed to have. He writes:

If it amuses anyone to assert this I cannot possibly refute him. But, on the other hand, there is not the least reason to believe him. If *any* memory-judgment be true, this one would seem to have the strongest possible claims. The numerical diversity of the two objective constituents is of course no bar to complete identity of their actual or their apparent qualities. And the two situations, and their respective objective constituents, are contiguous in time; so that there is the minimum possible opportunity for forgetting.[1]

Now though this reply may be satisfactory to the question of comparison via memory, I do not think that it meets the difficulty to which I have called attention with respect to Dr. Broad's remarks that sensa may have different qualities than we perceive them to have. The question which I am asking is: By what reason can we judge of a sensum already past that it had more or less or different characteristics than we perceived *it* as having, when all that we could ever inspect would be a subsequent and different objective constituent, which might very well be a numerically different sensum? To say that a given sensum was somehow different from the way it appeared to us to be would mean that the objective constituent of a *subsequent* visual situation had more or less or different characteristics than the objective constituent of the previous situation. To judge this, of course, we should have to depend on the accuracy of our memory, as Dr. Broad has said. Now though I quite readily accept with him the reliability of the relevant memory judgment of either similarity or difference, I cannot see that mere accuracy of memory alone would guarantee that the sensum perceived in the two pertinent visual situations was one and the same. And since the fact that sensum *b* was different from a preceding and numerically different sensum *a* would obviously not be evidence for the proposition that *a* had more or less or different characteristics than we perceived it as having, it is very important, if this proposition is to be meaningfully asserted, that the objective constituents of the two

[1] *Idem*, pp. 298 f.

pertinent visual situations be known to reveal one and the same sensum.

On Dr. Broad's own premises, however, I cannot see how this is possible. I am quite willing, as a matter of fact (for reasons which I will make clear in a moment), to concede that two *apparently identical* objective constituents reveal one and the same sensum— even though, on Dr. Broad's own argument, as I have said, the presumption would be against it, and there is nothing to prevent our holding that the objective constituents might 'really' be different in subtle and unnoticed ways, and hence might reveal numerically distinct sensa. But when the two objective constituents *differ* from each other in the characteristics which they appear to us to have, I cannot see that this concession can justifiably be made. If the objective constituent of the second (inspective) visual situation appears to have a more differentiated shape (e.g., ellipticity) than that which the objective constituent of the original visual situation appeared to have (e.g., circularity), then it seems to me that not only can we not know that they reveal one and the same sensum, but, on the contrary, this is good reason for holding that they do not. The very fact that the second sensum appeared to have the characteristic of ellipticity, while the first appeared to have the characteristic of circularity, would justify taking the view that they are not one and the same sensum. For what means is there of determining whether two temporally distinct perceptions are of two different sensa or of one and the same sensum, other than the perceptible differences or similarities between them? (This is why I think that it must be conceded —if one is going to entertain the notion of sensa at all—that *apparently identical* objective constituents reveal one and the same sensum.)

I think I have shown, then, that there is no sense in the assertion that a given sensum may have qualities which someone may have failed to notice. For there is not even a theoretically possible means of determining that a sensum is or was different from the way it appeared. And a difference that is not even theoretically capable of being detected is not a difference at all. Thus, so far as can be ascertained—and hence, so far as the limits of meaningful discourse allow—every sensum must have the characteristics it appears to have. There can be no significant distinction, with respect to sensa, between 'appearance' and 'reality'.

THE SENSUM THEORY

4

Now I think that the argument of the last section constitutes nothing less than a *reductio ad absurdum* of the Sensum Theory. And I want to make this clear.

The situation we have is this. The Sensum Theory holds that what we see 'directly'—i.e., the 'objective constituents' of our visual situations—are never literally parts of the surfaces of physical objects, but objects in their own right, namely sensa. The evidence on which the Theory rests consists of precisely the kind of facts that it was specifically designed to meet, viz., that the objective constituents of visual situations appear to have characteristics discrepant with those which we attribute to the physical objects we suppose ourselves to be seeing 'directly', the argument being that the objective constituents cannot hence be literally parts of the surfaces of these objects. Now it is clear that evidence which showed only that the objective constituents of a few perceptual situations have discrepant properties would leave practically unscathed the fundamental common-sense notion of an external world of physical objects directly revealed in sense-perception. In the way of this kind of evidence, then—which, so far as Dr. Broad has shown, is the only kind of evidence that could possibly establish the Sensum Theory—clearly what is required is a demonstration that the objective constituents of most if not all perceptual situations have perceptibly discrepant characteristics.

Unfortunately for Dr. Broad's argument, however, he is obliged, as we have seen, to come to terms with the fact that we do not 'as a rule'—in truth, in the vast majority of cases—perceive such discrepancies in our objective constituents: while the objective constituent of the visual situation when we look at a penny from a slightly oblique perspective admittedly may at first glance appear to be circular, he argues, 'more careful inspection' would reveal the objective constituent actually to be slightly elliptical in character. It is understandable, for one thing, he explains, that we should fail to notice a slight variation in curvature; but furthermore,

. . . we are not as a rule interested in sensa, as such, but only in what we think they can tell us about physical objects, which alone can help us or hurt us. Sensa themselves 'cut no ice'. We therefore pass automatically from the sensum and its properties to judgments about the physical object and its properties. If it should happen that the sensum is queer, as when we see double, we notice the sensum, as we notice an inverted letter. And, even in normal cases, we generally can detect the properties of sensa, and contrast them with those which they are leading us to ascribe to the physical object, *provided that we make a special effort of attention.*[1]

Thus it is clear that the tenability of the Sensum Theory hinges on the possibility of showing in this way that the objective constituents of our perceptual situations are actually different from the way they appear to us 'at first glance', on casual observation. Unless this is at least theoretically possible, not only would Dr. Broad be unable to meet a very cogent objection to the Sensum Theory, but by the same token, it must be appreciated, the very evidence necessary to establish even a *prima facie* case for the Theory against the common-sense notion would be theoretically impossible to achieve.

This brings us to the point of the discussion in the preceding section. The fact is that on Dr. Broad's way of analysing perception, 'showing a given objective constituent to be actually different from the way it appears to us at first glance' is simply not a significant possibility. For in order for this to be possible, it would have to be possible for us to know that we were taking a 'second look' at one and the same objective constituent, or else to know that 'careful inspection' of one objective constituent revealed anything about the characteristics of another. But on Dr. Broad's view that all we ever perceive 'directly', the objective constituents of our perceptual situations, are 'momentary, fleeting particulars', it is theoretically impossible for us to know either of these things.

In the first place, as we saw, Dr. Broad explicitly states that it is extremely doubtful that 'what we inspect' could ever be the same as 'what we perceive with'. And this means that he is conceding that any objective constituent about which we discover by a 'special effort of attention' or 'careful inspection' that it has discrepant characteristics is most probably a numerically different one from that about which we had noticed nothing peculiar. But whether or not Dr. Broad is right in his conviction that even ideally we could never simultaneously inspect and 'perceive with' numerically the same objective constituent, the unquestionable fact remains that we do not 'as a rule' perceive the peculiarities of our objective constituents, and cannot generally do so, as he admits, without

[1] *Scientific Thought*, p. 247 (italics mine).

'special effort of attention' and 'careful inspection'. And this means that for the great majority of cases, at any rate, the objective constituents about which we could perceive the peculiarities he describes would *in fact* have to be the objective constituents of *subsequent* (even if immediately succeeding) visual situations—subsequent, that is, to those which were not 'at *first* glance' perceived to have discrepant objective constituents, and which therefore must be capable of being shown to have actually had them, if a plausible case for the universal truth of the Sensum Theory is to be made. And with respect now to both this point and the preceding one, we take our cue from Dr. Broad's own argument concerning the problem of 'the external reference of our objective constituents' (cf. Chapters II and II, *supra*) and ask: What assurance is there that temporally distinct visual situations reveal one and the same objective constituent, or that temporally distinct objective constituents can be identified with 'a single, enduring and unchanging entity'—as would have to be the case for a 'second look' to be of any relevance or value? Or, to put the question more generally, what assurance is there that the objective constituent of a visual situation at time t_2 reveals anything about the objective constituents of visual situations at times t_1 or t_3?

On the common-sense view that what we see are relatively permanent and publicly inspectable physical objects, there would of course be no difficulty. In order to show that there are peculiarities about the appearances which physical objects present from different perspectives and under different conditions of observation, it would be relevant, for example, to appeal to causal considerations, such as the fact that when a circular coin is viewed from an oblique perspective the area of the retina affected by the light from the coin is an oblique projection of a circle, and must therefore be an ellipse. And on the strength of this, or in any case (since there is no question of continuous identity if the objective constituent is literally part of the kind of thing a physical object is conceived to be), we could relevantly be asked to attend more closely and thus perhaps achieve that degree of detachment necessary to see that the circular coin does indeed bear some resemblance, from an oblique perspective, to an ellipse—say to another coin mechanically distorted to the degree of ellipticity appropriate to that perspective—looked at from straight above.

But of course Dr. Broad insists that he does not *know* these things, since all that we ever perceive directly are 'transitory particulars'. And so if he is to demonstrate, as he must, that the objective constituents of most perceptual situations actually have discrepant characteristics even though we do not at first glance notice that they do, he is faced with the problem of showing in some other way that the objective constituent of one visual situation is numerically identical with or at least evidentially related to the objective constituent of another. For him simply to *assume* this would not do, of course. It would be an egregious piece of special pleading, in which the Sensum Theory would be allowed precisely the kind of assumption that he denies, as we have seen, to those who would defend the common-sense view. But for Dr. Broad to *show* on his own view that the characteristics of one objective constituent are relevant evidence for those of another obviously would require that he somehow 'transcend' the *phenomenal* world of sensa and establish the fact of such relevance from the vantage point of God in the *noumenal* world. And he has not given any evidence of being able to do this.

For all that Dr. Broad can show on his view, then, 'second looks', 'more careful inspections', or 'special efforts of attention' may very well always reveal an *independent* objective constituent, from whose properties, whether discrepant or not, nothing can be inferred with respect to any other objective constituent. And hence he cannot legitimately appeal to such means to establish that even when they do not seem to us to be so, the characteristics of the objective constituents of our perceptual situations are actually at variance with those we ascribe to the physical objects which we think we see. But if this essential evidence is beyond achievement, then so far as he can show to the contrary, the objective constituents of the vast majority of visual situations may very well be, as they seem, descriptively and numerically identical with the immediately visible surfaces of physical objects.

5

In the two sections immediately preceding I have tried to show that the Sensum Theory could not in any case be a satisfactory theory, because of the paradox that its consistent application would imply that we could not have known the vast majority of the very facts which it is supposed to explain and which constitute its sole possible evidence. Quite apart from this essentially formal argument, however, there are also certain more fundamental considerations, of a semantic nature, which show that the Sensum Theory, like the Multiple Inherence Theory and the Multiple Relation Theory, already discussed, is not a factually significant theory or hypothesis at all. And I want now briefly to present these considerations.

As we saw in Chapter IV, the Multiple Inherence Theory and the Multiple Relation Theory are purely *verbal* 'solutions' to Dr. Broad's pseudo-problem concerning the multiple appearances which physical objects present from different perspectives and under different conditions. They do not even deserve to be called *ad hoc* hypotheses. For as the term is commonly understood, an '*ad hoc* hypothesis' is one which invents a distinct entity or process to account for a given phenomenon; while to the undeniable phenomenon of the multiple appearances of physical objects the two 'theories', stripped of their technical jargon, do no more, as we saw, than give their formal consent, the first in effect merely allowing that the characteristics of physical objects may appear different to different simultaneous observers, or to the same observer from different vantage points, and the second that a physical object may appear (under certain conditions) to have characteristics that it does not actually have.

The Sensum Theory, on the other hand, in so far as it posits the existence of 'sensa', does seem at first glance to be at least an *ad hoc* hypothesis. Faced with the fact that objects look different under different circumstances, the Sensum Theory 'explains' it by the simple expedient of hypostatizing these 'appearances' into 'sensa', things in their own right, each one having precisely those characteristics appropriate to the circumstances in which it is seen, there being, of course, as many such 'things' as there are appearances to be accounted for. That this 'solution' is likewise no more than verbal, however, should be appreciated when it is recalled that these suppositious entities are *ex hypothesi* 'neither physical nor mental'. For so defined they are neatly extricated from the very possibility of independent and unambiguous verification or disverification. No amount of psychological, neurological, or physical investigation could ever establish their existence in perceptual situations, either 'in our minds', our brains, our eyes, or in the 'external world', as separate, numerically distinct entities, apart from what we unquestioningly take to be the immediately visible surfaces of physical objects. And thus, since 'sensa' are not distinguishable by appearance either, being, after all, descriptively identical with just those various different aspects or 'looks' which physical objects themselves are supposed to present—on the so-called 'common-sense view'—as the angle and other conditions causally relevant to their perception vary, it should be clear that no factual significance attaches to the 'hypothesis' that what we see directly are 'sensa' *rather than* the visible surfaces of physical objects. For a difference that is not even ideally capable of being discerned, either numerically or descriptively, is a difference in name alone.

It must be borne in mind, moreover, that whether the things we perceive 'directly' are called 'sensa' or 'physical objects', we still require, for practical as well as intellectual reasons, a coherent account or 'explanation' of the differences and similarities between what we perceive at one moment, under one set of conditions, and what we perceive at earlier and later moments, under specifiably different conditions; and also between our own perceptual experiences and those of others. On the so-called 'common-sense view', as we have seen, the differences and similarities between the various appearances presented by a physical object viewed from different vantage points and under different conditions are explained causally, in terms of our knowledge of such matters as the nature of light, geometric perspective, and the human perceptual apparatus. Now in the first place, however he might choose to describe it, the Sensum Theory adherent can hardly deny the efficacy of this knowledge, achieved and formulated in terms of the 'common-sense view', in enabling us to anticipate and influence empirical phenomena, and indeed, in enabling us to achieve *additional* such knowledge from which *further* successful prediction and control can result. But what is more important, it should be clear from the argument of the preceding paragraph that the Sensum Theory cannot of itself lead to any unambiguous consequences or verifiable predictions that are distinguishable from those which we are either already acquainted with or which we could equally well deduce and formulate, entirely in terms of the 'common-sense view'. Hence, obviously, if the adherent of the Sensum Theory is to be able to describe the multiplicity of phenomena coherently, and to provide us with a means of prediction and control such as we already enjoy, he must of necessity take account, in one form or another, of the whole body of this actual and possible common-sense knowledge. And in point of fact, it is perfectly apparent that Dr. Broad has done no more than just this, systematically translating into the formulas of the Sensum Theory the observable facts and predictive explanations which we already know in common-sense terms.

Thus the situation amounts to this: Call the succession of different appearances which an object presents as we walk about and observe it from different perspectives and under different conditions 'direct perceptions of the same physical object', and Dr. Broad finds himself unable to explain their similarities and differences; merely call them 'sensa', however, and though not even an ideally detectible further difference is involved, for him the difficulty at once subsides.

6

I want finally to explain the suggestion which I made in the first section of the present chapter that the real reason for Dr. Broad's preference for the Sensum Theory over the other two he proposes is to be found in his analysis of perception. Now the arguments of this and preceding chapters have shown the purely verbal character of all three of Dr. Broad's 'solutions' to his 'logical problem' concerning the different appearances which physical objects present under different conditions of observation; and they have also shown that these 'solutions' are in any event gratuitous, since the fact of the multiple appearances can be adequately explained scientifically, in terms wholly compatible with our common-sense notions about physical objects and perception. And thus in itself the discussion of Dr. Broad's preferences for one or another of his 'alternative theories' would be supererogatory. But I think that the present discussion will also serve to shed further light on a much more important question, with which I have dealt only superficially thus far: namely, just why it is that Dr. Broad cannot allow that the scientific, common-sense explanation satisfactorily reconciles the multiple appearances with the notion of a single, unchanging physical object 'directly revealed' in perception.

In the exposition of the 'logical question' and the alternative theories, in Chapter IV, it may be recalled, I noted Dr. Broad's comment that, were it not for the fact that we have to consider the possibility of a number of observers having simultaneous perceptions whose objective constituents were descriptively incompatible with each other, it might be *more reasonable* to adopt the alternative that a physical object is not of constant size and shape, as is commonly believed, but that it varies in these respects as the observer walks about, than to suppose that the objective constituent of a visual situation does not have some of the properties which it seems to have, and does have properties inconsistent with these.[1] I want to consider now just why Dr. Broad should find it *prima facie* more reasonable to suppose that a physical object is affected by or varies with the movements of an observer, than to allow that the objective constituent has properties different from those which it may appear to have in certain perceptual situations. As I have shown, the latter is, in fact, what we ordinarily do believe about perception and physical objects; and it is far more plausible to common sense than the former. For the former suggests a wholly unfamiliar and inexplicable type of situation, while illusory experience—especially the commonplace type to which Dr. Broad refers—is both familiar and readily explainable in terms of what we know of geometrical and physical optics and of the physiology of vision.

The reason for Dr. Broad's peculiar prejudice in this matter, I want to suggest, is that from the very outset he approaches the analysis of perception with a certain unfounded notion concerning the nature of the objective constituents of visual situations. I believe that he regards them from the first as something akin to the kind of 'entity' he has in mind when he employs the term 'sensum', and that this is why he is inclined to favour the Multiple Inherence Theory (and especially the Sensum Theory) over either the common-sense view or the more closely akin Multiple Relation Theory of Appearing, as solutions to the problem which he feels about the unique appearances which objects present from different perspectives. I want to try to show this.

Let us begin by assuming that Dr. Broad does mean by the term 'objective constituent', as he originally gives us to understand, simply what might be called the *descriptive content* of a visual experience—i.e., what the qualitative description of a visual hallucination would have in common with the qualitative

[1] *The Mind and Its Place in Nature*, p. 159.

description of a veridical visual perception, if both experiences seemed to reveal, say, a pink rat. Thus, in speaking of a pink rat as being the objective constituent of a visual situation, it would be an open question as to whether the objective constituent was literally an external physical object (or at least a spatio-temporal *part* of an external physical object), or whether the experience was merely hallucinatory, though qualitatively very much like that which we should have if we were actually to perceive such an animal. With this in mind, then, let us now consider the fact that Dr. Broad finds it *prima facie* unreasonable to suppose that the objective constituent of a visual situation might have qualities different from those which it appeared to have from a particular perspective.

Now when we consider an hallucinatory situation, it is not at all difficult to understand why Dr. Broad should hold this. It would simply make no sense to say that the objective constituent of an hallucinatory experience had qualities different from what it appeared to have. For that would be to treat the objective constituent of the hallucinatory experience as though it were a physical object having permanent intrinsic physical character-istics which could be subsequently determined as being other than as they were originally experienced; whereas, of course, in hallucinatory experience there is no such object. The objective constituent in visual hallucination (e.g., an after-image of a bright red light), bears somewhat the same type of relation to the subject of the experience and to the actual bright red light, as the throbbing which the recent amputee is commonly said to 'feel in the amputated limb' does to the amputee and to the absent limb. To say that the qualities of either of these experiences are 'really' different from the way they are experienced is obviously not to assert a meaningful possibility. Thus, with respect to the qualities of the objective constituents of hallucinatory experiences, it is clear that *esse est percipi.*

But Dr. Broad is disinclined to allow that even when the experience in question is not hallucinatory, the objective con-stituent could have characteristics other than it seemed to have. And here it is not at all clear why he should take this position. For if the objective constituent is allowed to be literally a spatio-temporal part of an external physical object, then it is supposed to have relatively permanent intrinsic physical characteristics;

and subsequent more careful inspection would be entirely relevant, and might very well reveal the object to have characteristics different from those which it appeared to have under certain conditions or from certain perspectives.

Dr. Broad's puzzle is how it could be that the objective constituent of a visual situation could 'really have' characteristics other than those which it seems 'on careful inspection' to have. Now, in the first place, it is well to note again that what we should ordinarily call 'careful inspection' of a physical object would involve looking at it from various perspectives, especially from straight above, handling it, measuring it, etc. But it is clear that Dr. Broad has in mind not the careful inspection of an object in this way, but only careful attention to the way the object looks from certain perspectives—e.g., the unique elliptical appearance which a penny presents from an oblique perspective. And hence, if Dr. Broad really means to allow that the objective constituent of the visual situation may literally be the external physical object itself, his puzzle, then, is not how the objective constituent could seem *on careful inspection* to have characteristics other than those which it actually has, but rather how it could seem when carefully inspected *from certain oblique perspectives* to have characteristics other than those which it actually has. The answer to this emended question is to be found, of course, in what we know of geometrical and physical optics and the physiology of vision. The visual perception of an object is a process which involves light reflection from the object to our eyes. Light travels in a more or less straight line; and hence we perceive the object in geometric perspective. When we look at a penny from the side, the light which reaches our eyes from the penny is an oblique projection of a circle, which is an ellipse; and so the round penny looks from the side somewhat the way an elliptical disc looks when viewed from straight above.

This answer, however, as we have seen, is not satisfactory to Dr. Broad. If *what we see* when we look at the penny from the side, the objective constituent of our visual situation, is elliptical, and the penny is supposed to be round, then how, he still insists, can the objective constituent be literally a spatio-temporal part of the penny? Dr. Broad is clearly not to be put off with the common-sense objection that *what we see* when we look at a penny from the side is the penny itself, and that, hence, *what we see* is round, and not elliptical. 'Words like "seeing" and "hearing" are hopeless for our present purposes if they are to be interpreted in this way', is Dr. Broad's reply to this, as we have seen. 'The plain fact', he insists, 'is that "looking elliptical to me" stands for a peculiar experience, which, whatever the right analysis of it may be, is not just a mistaken judgment about the shape of the penny.' And subsequently he remarks that 'When I look at a penny from the side I am certainly aware of *something*; and it is certainly plausible to hold that this something is elliptical in the same plain sense in which a suitable bent piece of wire, looked at from straight above, is elliptical."

Now from the fact that Dr. Broad's insistence that 'what we see' when we view a penny obliquely is elliptical is not to be appeased by the type of explanation which I have advanced in terms of the behaviour of light, etc., I am led to believe that Dr. Broad wants to *begin* by regarding the objective constituents of visual situations as something akin to what he understands by the term 'sensa', and *only then* to consider the question of whether or not, and if so how, objective constituents can be literally spatio-temporal parts of external physical objects. For in rejecting the type of explanation which I have given, he seems to be regarding the objective constituent *statically*, so to speak, as though it were a kind of object-in-its-own-right, apart from the penny, literally having the spatial outline of ellipticity, instead of *functionally*, as the penny itself seen via the oblique projection of the light from its surface.

It would seem that even though Dr. Broad is willing, in theory, to allow that the objective constituents of visual situations are not the unique kind of entities which he has in mind when he employs the term 'sensa', his conception of the objective constituent is that it is in any case a kind of two-dimensional visual 'picture', which, if not a sensum, is at least then a mental 'image'. On this view, that what we are 'immediately' aware of in visual experience are 'images', and never external physical objects 'directly', the difference between hallucination and normal perception is merely that in the latter case the 'image' is produced when the light from external physical objects impinges on the retina and activates the optic nerve and the occipital lobe of the brain, while in the former case it is internally produced. On the one hand, there is the external object, and on the other, there is the 'visual image', which, in ideal cases, merely 'corresponds' to the external object.

The foregoing, of course, is the familiar 'theory of representative ideas' which was advanced, in one form or another by such philosophers as Descartes, Hobbes, and Locke, and in more recent times by the Critical Realists. Now, to be sure, as I noted in the exposition of the Sensum Theory at the beginning of the present chapter, Dr. Broad says that the doctrine of representative ideas is only the 'traditional and highly muddled' form of the Sensum Theory. But it seems, in view of the preceding discussion, that the only real alternative to the Sensum Theory which he can conceive is some form of this 'representative' theory. For he does insist on treating the objective constituents of our visual situations as though they were separate and distinguishable pictorial representations which actually have the spatial properties which they seem to have, even though these properties may not correspond exactly to those which the external physical object actually has. And he refuses to accept a functional causal explanation for the unique appearances of objects from oblique perspectives—which is the only type of explanation, it seems to me, on which the objective constituent can properly be said to be directly and literally part of the surface of the penny itself. For if the objective constituent is conceived to be actually elliptical, in the same sense as the penny is actually round, then it is clear at the outset that whatever *rapprochement* be effected between the two, it cannot be that of literal, numerical identity.

If I am correct that Dr. Broad explicitly or implicitly holds some such notion about the objective constituent, even as he is considering the question of the relation of the objective constituent to the physical object, then I think it becomes understandable why he finds it unreasonable to suppose that the objective constituents of non-hallucinatory visual situations could have characteristics different from those which they seem to have. For then there is the same 'incorrigibility' that there is in the case of hallucinatory perception. If the objective constituents of veridical visual experiences are 'mental images', and not external physical objects, it would be as unreasonable to suppose that they could have characteristics other than those which they appear to have, as to suppose that a particular after-image is really different from the way it appears to the individual whose experience it is, or a pain different from the way it feels. On this view of the nature of objective constituents, moreover, 'careful inspection' of it does not mean examining the external physical object more closely, handling it, rotating it before one's eyes, measuring it, etc. Rather it means simply attending carefully to one's own momentary, private 'visual image'. For if the objective constituent is this sort of thing, every change of position on the part of the observer would produce a *different* objective constituent, a different 'image'. And hence, 'careful inspection' of a given objective constituent is limited to the single given perspective in which that particular objective constituent is revealed. There is no other perspective at all from which *that particular* image can be seen; and, *a fortiori*, there is no 'more ideal' vantage point from which to inspect it. Thus, it would be as inconceivable that one should be mistaken about the 'actual' qualities of the objective constituent of which he was directly aware, as it would, on the common-sense view, that he should be mistaken about the actual qualities of a penny which he had examined under the most ideal conditions. And now it also becomes clear why Dr. Broad should insist that considerations of perspective and the like are wholly irrelevant; for they are 'external' considerations, and cannot intervene between the individual's 'awareness' and the objective constituent, if the latter be conceived as his own 'private', 'immediate', 'visual image'.

I think I have shown, then, how it could be that Dr. Broad finds it *prima facie* unreasonable to suppose that the objective constituent of a visual situation could have characteristics different from those which it seems 'on careful inspection' to have. But I said at the outset of this discussion that in considering this it would also become clear why Dr. Broad should suppose that the different appearances which objects present from different perspectives constitute a problem at all. And I think that this is now also clear, in view of the foregoing.

What troubles Dr. Broad, I think, is something like this. Suppose we photographed a penny from an oblique perspective, and then cut out the photographic image of the penny with scissors. The result of this procedure would be an elliptical piece of photographic paper. And it is obvious that this elliptical piece of paper could not be placed flat on the surface of the penny in such a way that its outline would coincide exactly with the penny.

Now if Dr. Broad considers the objective constituent of the visual situation in which we see the penny from an oblique perspective, to be a kind of 'visual image', like the photographic image, only 'non-material', then it becomes understandable at once why he should find it so implausible to suppose that the objective constituent of this visual situation could be literally spatio-temporally identical with the surface of the round penny. It is as though he imagined the outcome of a procedure similar to that which I have described with respect to the photographic image, in which he would take a pair of fine tweezers and, ever so delicately, pick up the fragile, tenuous 'visual image' and lay it carefully over the face of the penny. As in the case of the photographic cut-out, it would obviously not coincide in outline with the penny itself. Thus, Dr. Broad is at a loss to understand how the objective constituent could possibly be held to be literally spatio-temporally identical with the surface of the penny.

On this view, then, Dr. Broad's concern is quite understandable. *If* when we looked at a penny from the side, an 'image' were produced (in our eyes? in our optic nerves? in our minds?), like a photographic image, distinct from the penny itself, and this were the objective constituent of our 'immediate' visual experience, then the objective constituent would not only not be *numerically* identical with the surface of the penny, it would not even be *descriptively* identical. Being an oblique projection of a circle, the 'image' would be elliptical. But, of course, this is just the issue: *is* the objective constituent a separate and distinguishable 'entity', having its own shape and size in the same sense as the penny does? For only if it is does the fact that objects present unique appearances from different points of observation constitute a problem. If it is not, and the objective constituents of the various perceptual situations are all simply different perspectual views of the one penny, then the fact that they differ from each other and from the limiting case in which the penny is viewed from straight above, is obviously accounted for by the fact that we see objects with our eyes, by means of the reflection of light. The behaviour of light and the nature of our eyes result, in a perfectly understandable way, in the familiar visual phenomena of perspectual distortion of size and shape. Thus, in order even to raise the problem of the incompatibility of the objective constituents with the one object, Dr. Broad has to assume from the start, without warrant, that they are separate and distinct 'entities' having their own size and shape in the same sense in which the physical object does. And in doing this he begs the question. For he obviously cannot regard the objective constituent as a kind of photographic image, literally having the geometric characteristic of ellipticity, and remain neutral with respect to the question of whether it is or is not literally spatio-temporally identical with the surface of the penny which literally has the geometric characteristic of circularity.

7

We have seen, then, that Dr. Broad must begin his analysis of perception with some such implicit notion about 'objective constituents' as he later explicitly favours in espousing the Sensum Theory, and that this accounts both for the problem he feels and the solution he favours. Now I believe that this conception of the 'objective constituents' of perceptual experience as distinct *entities* which literally have qualities and spatial characteristics 'in the same plain sense' in which physical objects do, and which stand to 'external' physical objects in somewhat the same relation that photographic images do, is a confusion to which Dr. Broad's sense-datum approach to the analysis of perception is peculiarly susceptible. And I want briefly, in concluding the essay, to suggest how it comes about.

Let us to begin with remember what the sense-datum approach involves. As we have seen in Chapter I and subsequently, Dr. Broad does not wish to deny that we do from time to time have such perceptual experiences as are commonly indicated by expressions like 'I see a chair', 'I see a bell', 'I hear a bell', etc. But he is concerned about the relation of whatever it is that we are 'directly aware of' in such experiences—i.e., our 'sense-data' or 'objective constituents'—to the 'external physical objects' we claim to be perceiving. Were it not, he says, for the existence of illusions and hallucinations, there would be no grounds for questioning whether this relation is what it seems to be, namely, one of literal, descriptive and numerical identity. But the existence of such aberrant experiences, he feels, obliges us to re-examine this relationship and our notions about physical objects in general.

THE SENSUM THEORY

Now I have already argued at some length, in Chapter III particularly, that the fact of occasional delusive perceptual situations does not in the first place call for any such drastic re-examination as Dr. Broad thinks necessary, and that it cannot in any event support his startling conclusions with respect to *all* perceptual experience. And I shall not repeat those arguments here. My concern here is rather to show the pitfall inherent in the position Dr. Broad adopts in carrying out his enterprise, a pitfall, as I shall try to make clear, which foredooms the investigation to the paradoxical conclusions at which he ultimately arrives.

In raising the question Dr. Broad, as we have seen, proposes to take what he regards as a neutral position with respect to all sensory experience. That is, he wants to begin by regarding all sensory experience which purports to be perceptual, whether it be in the ordinary sense hallucinatory or veridical, as though it were hallucinatory, like a 'dream-image', or an 'after-image'; and then afterwards to distinguish those experiences, if there be any, which can be determined to be 'directly' revelatory of external physical objects. But to begin by considering all perceptual experience in abstraction, apart from physical objects, turns out not to be quite so 'neutral' a procedure as it seems at first consideration to be. For it is this very approach to his quest, I think, that is responsible for Dr. Broad's apparent predisposition to conceive the 'objective constituents' of all perceptual experience as objects in their own right, having qualities and properties in the same sense that physical objects do, which, as we saw in the preceding section, is at the bottom of his 'logical problem'. And I want now to show how the sense-datum approach predisposes to this question-begging conception.

To begin with, I want to draw attention to the obvious fact that our ordinary, non-philosophical mode of thinking and speaking about sensible qualities and properties derives from normal perceptual experience in which the particular colours, shapes, etc., of which we are aware are the sensible qualities and properties of physical objects immediately present to our senses. There are, to be sure, non-veridical experiences in which this is not the case. But for the most part, certainly, we have no difficulty in predicating particular qualities and properties, such as brownness, roundness, and the like, of particular publicly identifiable physical objects. And hence the conception is firmly ingrained in our thought

204

and speech that such predicates have appropriate *substantives* whose predicates they are; and that what we perceive when we perceive these qualities and properties are these substantives.

Now this substantive-predicate mode of thought and speech would occasion no difficulty were it not for the fact of hallucinations and hallucinatory-like experiences—e.g., dreams and after-images—in which we are aware of particular qualities and characteristics which we know are not the qualities or characteristics of external objects present to our senses at the moment. For this is when the substantive-predicate habit of thought and speech, so useful in ordinary cases, proves to be a source of confusion. Instead of simply recognizing such experiences as pathological internal disturbances of our sensory apparatus, our eyes, nervous system, and brain, giving rise to sensory experiences which are like those we have when we see physical objects via external stimulation of our eyes, we still want—at least in discourse—to attribute the qualities which constitute these subjective experiences, to a substantive. And since it does not make any sense to say that it is our *sensations* which are literally brown, or round, etc., we adopt a peculiar linguistic device. We speak of 'visual patches': thus, 'square *patch* of red'; or else, more commonly, as in the case of after-imaging, we say that it is our *after-image* which is red and square. To be sure, we may employ these expressions without necessarily believing that 'patches' and 'after-images' are *things*. Nevertheless, the use of such terms does preserve the substantive-predicate mode of speech; and this tends to cause us to conceive of our after-sensations as though they were a peculiar kind of *entity*, 'immediately present to our minds', in which the qualities and characteristics of our pathological sensations 'inhere'. Because we conceive of them as 'immediate' and 'mental', however, they present no scientific difficulties; and thus, safe from empirical refutation, we trouble ourselves no further.

Let us see now how a similar situation arises in the course of Dr. Broad's sense-datum approach to the analysis of perceptual experience. This approach we have seen involves regarding the 'objective constituents' of perceptual situations in abstraction, apart from the physical objects which we are not, at least at the outset, supposed to know exist. But now, when he does this, Dr. Broad, it must be borne in mind, is locking himself in from without; and this is the source of the difficulty. What I mean is this. Before he undertakes the sense-datum type of analysis, Dr. Broad is of course as much aware as anyone else that there are such things as we ordinarily understand by the term 'physical object', and that such things have various qualities and properties, like brownness and roundness. Hence he too has the substantive-predicate conception firmly ingrained in his thought and speech. And thus even when he considers our perceptual sensations in abstraction he still wants to attribute the qualities and properties of which we are aware to some substantive. Inasmuch as he is supposing that we do not know that there are such things, or that they are 'directly revealed' in sensory experience, however, he cannot allow that this substantive is a physical object. And since, again, it does not seem to make any sense to say that it is a *sensation* which is literally round, brown, etc., Dr. Broad, like the naïve person in the case of after-images, implicitly regards the 'objective constituent' as a kind of photographic image which literally has these properties and qualities in the same sense that physical objects do.

Now of course it matters little if the ordinary individual eases his troubled metaphysical conscience with some such device in speaking about hallucinatory experience. But it is quite another matter when a metaphysically inclined empiricist like Dr. Broad is likewise victimized by this desire for verbal and conceptual symmetry. For then it gives rise to all sorts of nagging puzzles. Thus, as we have seen, it permits Dr. Broad to generate a 'logical problem' out of the familiar, scientifically explicable fact that an object looks different under different conditions of observation. And in consequence the issue is subtly transformed from that of whether or not the 'objective constituent' is literally an 'external physical object', or at least the immediately perceptible surface of one, to that of whether it can be somehow *linked* with a 'larger external whole'. And, of course, inevitably the question arises: if what we are 'immediately aware of' in perceptual sensation are merely 'objective constituents', or 'sense-data', how, then, can we possibly know that there are such things as 'external physical objects'?

To be sure, after the problem is set in these terms, Dr. Broad is willing to discuss the possibility that the 'objective constituents' of our perceptual experiences may be literally part of the 'external physical objects' which we 'seem to see'. But unfortunately this will not work. For once the verbal separation is made, between '*private*' objective constituents or sense-data, and '*public*' physical objects, it is impossible to reunite the two in any logically justified way, as Dr. Broad well recognizes. Thus the moral is clear: if one wants to avoid the 'logical problem' and the whole pseudo-problem about 'our knowledge of the external world', which can lead only to Dr. Broad's sceptical conclusions and paradoxical 'theories', one must be careful not to be trapped by the apparently innocent but actually unresolvable verbal separations of the sense-datum approach, in the first place.

> 'He strikes no coin, 'tis true, but coins
>   new phrases,
> And vends them forth as knaves vend
>   gilded counters,
> Which wise men scorn, and fools accept
>   in payment.'
>
> (Scott, *The Monastery*)

BIBLIOGRAPHY
(TEXTUAL REFERENCES)

BROAD, C. D., 'Critical and Speculative Philosophy', in *Contemporary British Philosophy* (First Series), edited by J. H. Muirhead, London, Allen & Unwin, 1924, pp. 75–100.

Examination of McTaggart's Philosophy, Cambridge, Cambridge University Press, Vol. 1, 1933, Vol. 2, 1938.

The Mind and Its Place in Nature, London, Kegan Paul, 1925.

Perception, Physics, and Reality, Cambridge, Cambridge University Press, 1914.

Scientific Thought, London, Kegan Paul, 1923.

MOORE, G. E., 'A Defence of Common Sense', in *Contemporary British Philosophy* (Second Series), edited by J. H. Muirhead, London, Allen & Unwin, 1925, pp. 193–223.

'The Nature of Sensible Appearances' (Symposium with G. Dawes Hicks, H. H. Price, and L. Stebbing), *Aristotelian Society, Suppl. Vol. VI*, 1926, pp. 142–205 (Moore's contribution: pp. 179–89).

'The Refutation of Idealism', *Mind*, Vol. 12, Oct. 1903, pp. 433–53.

'A Reply to My Critics', in *The Philosophy of G. E. Moore* (The Library of Living Philosophers), edited by P. A. Schilpp, Evanston and Chicago, Northwestern University Press, 1942, pp. 533–677.

PRICE, H. H., *Perception*, New York, McBride, 1933.

RUNES, D. D., ed., *Dictionary of Philosophy*, New York, Philosophical Library, 1942.

RUSSELL, B. A. W., *The Analysis of Mind*, London, Allen & Unwin, 1921.

Mysticism and Logic and Other Essays, London, Longmans, Green, 1918.

Our Knowledge of the External World, New York, Norton, 1929.

The Problems of Philosophy, New York, Holt, 1912.

BIBLIOGRAPHY

STEBBING, L. S., *Philosophy and the Physicists*, London, Methuen, 1938.

WISDOM, J. T., 'Moore's Technique', in *The Philosophy of G. E. Moore* (The Library of Living Philosophers), edited by P. A. Schilpp, Evanston and Chicago, Northwestern University Press, 1942, pp. 419–50.

'Other Minds', *Mind*, Vols. 49–52, 1940–43.

WITTGENSTEIN, L., *Tractatus Logico-Philosophicus*, London, Kegan Paul, 1922.

INDEX

(See also the synopsis of chapters, *Introduction*, pp. 28–33.)

INDEX

INDEX

INDEX

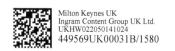
Milton Keynes UK
Ingram Content Group UK Ltd.
UKHW022050141024
449569UK00031B/1580